HEALTHCARE ECONOMICS
MADE EASY

HEALTHCARE ECONOMICS
MADE EASY

DANIEL JACKSON

Research Fellow in Health Economics,
University of Surrey

Scion

© Scion Publishing Ltd 2012

ISBN 978 1 904842 94 1

A CIP catalogue record for this book is available from the British Library.

Scion Publishing Limited
The Old Hayloft, Vantage Business Park, Bloxham Road, Banbury,
Oxfordshire OX16 9UX

www.scionpublishing.com

Important Note from the Publisher

The information contained within this book was obtained by Scion Publishing Limited from sources believed by us to be reliable. However, while every effort has been made to ensure its accuracy, no responsibility for loss or injury whatsoever occasioned to any person acting or refraining from action as a result of information contained herein can be accepted by the authors or publishers.

Although every effort has been made to ensure that all owners of copyright material have been acknowledged in this publication, we would be pleased to acknowledge in subsequent reprints or editions any omissions brought to our attention.

Readers should remember that medicine is a constantly evolving science and while the authors and publishers have ensured that all dosages, applications and practices are based on current indications, there may be specific practices which differ between communities. You should always follow the guidelines laid down by the manufacturers of specific products and the relevant authorities in the country in which you are practising.

Typeset by Techastra Solutions (P) Ltd.
Printed and bound in Great Britain by 4edge Ltd, Hockley. www.4edge.co.uk

Contents

Preface

This book is designed for healthcare professionals and managers who need a basic understanding of the world of health economics and health economic evaluation, but don't have the desire to become health economists.

Whether the thought of conducting an economic evaluation leaves you feeling queasy, or just plain confused, sometimes we all need to be able to understand why certain treatments have been chosen over other alternatives. To do this we need a working understanding of the methods and techniques a health economist like me uses every day. You **don't** need to be able to build a complicated economic model, or to understand all the mathematics which can often go with these analyses, but you do need to understand the **approach** health economists have taken to reach these conclusions.

This book does not assume that you have any previous experience with health economics. Even if the only economic decision you've ever made is from shopping on the high street, you will find that everything here is clearly laid out and explained.

The 'star' system has been designed to help you to go straight to the most important concepts if you are in a hurry.

I have also rated each of the concepts for how easy it is to understand. Sometimes, some aspects of health economics are very straightforward, while others may be very confusing first time around. I suggest you build up to some of the more complex concepts in your own time.

Honestly, once you have a good understanding of these approaches, you'll never stop thinking like an economist!

Daniel Jackson

January 2012

Acknowledgements

Huge thanks to my editors Simon and Jonathan for their tireless work on this and for always believing in the project. I especially thank them for making sure that I don't write like an economist! Thanks also goes to Clare at Scion Publishing for reading the early draft from cover to cover, a task far beyond the call of duty!

I also have to thank my family, but most of all I say thank you to my beautiful wife Anna and wonderful son Dylan, who have to live with an economist every single day. Thank you for always understanding.

1 Health economics
...and why you need to know about it.

Economics is simply the science of scarcity. There just isn't enough to go round. Ever. So economists try to develop and implement a system which enables tough choices to be made and in doing so, hopefully improve the lot of most of the people, most of the time. That includes you.

The field of health economics is all about applying those same economic tools and ideas to the world of healthcare, as generally speaking there isn't enough healthcare to go around either. Unfortunately, this also includes you.

Now, most people don't like wasting their money. Nothing hurts more than buying something only to watch it break, or fail as soon as you take it out of the box. Specifically, we all want 'value for money'. This is the goal of the health economist. The health economist wants to be able to help a healthcare professional deliver value for money services, or to avoid investing in something which doesn't provide value for money. So, how do we get the maximum value for money for the health service, hospital or patient?

Let's just take a quick step back here… What do we actually mean when we say we want 'value for money'? This concept, whilst intuitive to most people, can have a number of slightly different meanings depending on the context in which it is used. Often people may say 'value for money' when they acquire what they want, at the least cost.

EXAMPLE 1.1 VALUE FOR MONEY?

'My car was great value for money. It was only £500.' Now, we've all said something similar, but we know deep down this statement isn't always correct, nor is it always the best way to look at things.

- What if the cheaper car breaks down more often than the alternative?
- What if it didn't have all the features you really wanted?
- What if it actually cost more to run?

Some people refer to this idea as 'false economy'. You've focused purely on the price, and not taken into account the 'true' costs of the choice you've made. It may well be that over the long term the £500 car will cost far more than a car which cost £1000.

So, 'value for money' can be a tricky concept. Almost always we do need to think about more than just the price tag. We have to evaluate what we are actually purchasing, its purpose, and how long we are going to be using it for. To use economic language, we need to think about the long-term **benefits** of the product, and more formally, we need to think about the '**cost-effectiveness**' of the purchase.

I've no doubt that you will have heard of economists using an associated idea, that of **efficiency**. This is a measure of how well a resource is used in order to achieve an outcome. We'll talk more about this idea later, but crudely, if something is cost-effective it really helps if it is efficient too.

One of the simplest ideas in economics is that of **opportunity cost**, but more often than not this idea is not easily understood. I was lucky as I was introduced to this concept from a very early age; my father always used to give me my pocket money and say 'Remember, you can only spend it once'. This is the perfect example of opportunity cost thinking. If the young me wanted to buy that bar of chocolate, well I could, but it would mean that I would not be able to buy the bottle of pop I also wanted, as I could only spend my pocket money once. So the opportunity cost of the chocolate bar is the bottle of pop. It's what we have forgone when making our decisions. Today, my opportunity cost trade-offs are 'Should I have a new car or a holiday this year?' If I choose to go on holiday, the opportunity cost of the holiday is the new car I now can't afford.

In health economics, this idea makes clear the very real trade-offs that managers and clinicians have to make when allocating resources for use within the health services. The true cost of using scarce healthcare funding to provide a service is their unavailability to fund an alternative healthcare service which would also be beneficial.

I hope you are starting to see that we are all economists; you just don't fully recognize it yet, but you will! All economic evaluations have a simple common structure which you already know. It is the assessment of what we spend to achieve or attain something ('costs') and the outcomes of this action ('benefits').

Here's an example from a typical Saturday for me. I'm thirsty. Should I buy a coffee on the high street now, and have a coffee quickly but pay quite a lot for it, or should I just wait until I get home, and have a cheaper coffee, but stay thirsty for longer? Without really thinking about it I am simply weighing up the costs (higher price of immediate coffee) against the benefits (quenched thirst), and then coming to a decision. Normally I'll end up buying the coffee. The key point here, though, is that we all do this type of instinctive economic analysis over almost every purchase, only economists tend to realize we're doing it.

So when thinking about health economics, you can see that an economic approach can help to inform and hopefully improve any decision-making in healthcare through the systematic and objective application of economic tools which, if we're brutally honest, is sometimes just 'common sense'.

However, 'common sense' is not always that easy to find, which is why frameworks for this type of analysis have been built to enable us to fully balance the costs and benefits of a decision. This allows us to be more confident in our decisions and is an invaluable mode of thinking for all healthcare professionals, irrespective of whether or not a full, formal economic evaluation is undertaken.

So, we now know that economics is the science of choosing. We have to make choices simply because we don't have unlimited resources. Formally, economics analyses how these choices are considered and ultimately prioritized, to generate the greatest welfare benefit within the context of clearly constrained resources.

We also now know that we all, subconsciously or not, use economics on a daily basis ('Do I buy the cheaper car, or pay a bit more for the nicer one?') as we live every day within our own budgets (my heart says, 'Buy the nicer one'; my head says, 'Buy the cheaper one'). By clearly comparing the true costs and benefits associated with the purchase of the alternative cars, we are able to rationalize, and hopefully improve, our decisions.

That said, we must also acknowledge that the world of healthcare is different. It isn't quite the same as choosing between cars, or chocolate bars. Healthcare technologies often have special characteristics that affect such analyses. How can we value a treatment which would allow someone to not be wheelchair-bound for the rest of their life? Can we compare this with the value of someone not going blind? This is what I believe makes health economics so interesting and vital.

Health economists try to capture that universal desire to eke out the maximum value for money from the healthcare budget, by ensuring not just that the healthcare interventions or technologies actually have a therapeutic value and are effective, but also that these interventions are a truly cost-effective proposition.

It is widely known that healthcare systems across the world don't have the means to be able to provide all of the new, complex and expensive health technologies which are available. The health needs of the population invariably exceed the budgets and funding of all the different healthcare systems in the world today. Once we understand and accept that healthcare decision-makers have to make difficult choices, we need to think about how we inform those choices and ultimately prioritize some health interventions over other interventions through the comparison of their total costs and their true benefits.

So, the aim of this book is to give you the tools to make, and understand, health economics decisions. As I demonstrated above, if we regularly make use of such economic techniques, even without knowing it, every day, then surely we should be able to apply these ideas formally? Perhaps you are a health professional today or hope to be one in the future, or are simply interested in the field of health economics. Wherever you are coming from, the concepts presented above are the cornerstone of health economic evaluation, and this book will guide you through the techniques health economists use every single day. But believe me, they are never far from the fundamental ideas we've just gone through!

2 Thinking like an economist

The following chapters in this book go into detail about the various analyses and techniques used in health economics and used in the economic evaluation of healthcare technologies. However, and in particular if you are new to this subject, I would recommend you spend a bit a time reading and re-reading this chapter so that you can start to understand how an economist thinks.

As we said in *Chapter 1*, healthcare economics is really all about how we decide to allocate scarce resources (budgets, time, people, etc.) in a way that achieves the very best healthcare outcomes possible.

So, let's start with an example of a healthcare decision and work through this as a healthcare economist might:

> ### EXAMPLE 2.1 WONDERLEVE
>
> A new drug – we'll call it Wonderleve – has just been launched for the treatment of migraine.
>
> It's more expensive than our existing treatment – known as Average-aid – but the clinical data suggest that it works a lot better too.
>
> So, should we decide to prescribe Wonderleve for all migraine sufferers, instead of Average-aid?
>
> How would a health economist approach this decision? And what would they be taking into consideration?

Health outcomes

The first thing a health economist would do would be to look at the impact each treatment has on **health outcomes**.

So what do we mean when we talk of a 'health outcome'?

We cannot make a true evaluation of any healthcare intervention without a measure of the benefit we are buying – in this case, the impact of the treatment on a person's health.

This is where health economics really starts to get interesting (well, I think it does!). Actually sitting down and defining just what a health outcome is, and then trying to consistently measure it is not easy, to say the least. You may think that in our example, 'not having a migraine' is the health outcome we're looking at, but there is often more to consider than just this type of measure…

Health outcomes are often defined in terms of people living longer. You can think of this as 'adding years to life'. Alongside this concept is the idea of improving someone's quality of life (QoL) as a health outcome; this can be thought of as 'adding life to years'. Some people would say they would prefer a shorter healthy life than a long one plagued by illness.

Surprisingly, there are many measures which are used to assess the impact of a healthcare intervention on survival. Researchers use ideas such as lives saved, or life years gained, or five-year survival rates. All are great measures and all have a place but, in my experience, decision-makers are starting to think more about the impact an intervention has on a patient's overall quality of life.

Improved quality of life is a complex idea, because many things can affect a person's quality of life. In *Example 2.1*, reduced migraine pain would certainly improve the patient's quality of life; in addition, if the new treatment Wonderleve allows migraine sufferers to resume their normal activities much sooner than Average-aid does, then we should also include measures of mobility – perhaps the ability of the patient to do their job, to socialize, and even their emotional wellbeing.

So health economists usually try to combine all of these elements in one measure: **health-related quality of life** (HRQoL). We will discuss this in more detail in *Chapter 5*.

When we have a value for the quality of life, we then aim to combine it with the quantity of life generated by the treatment. I won't go into all of the details here, as we will discuss this further in *Chapters 6 and 7*. A result of this kind of work is a measure you will almost certainly have heard of – the QALY or Quality-Adjusted Life Year.

The QALY approach involves applying weights to the clinical outcomes a treatment confers that reflect the preferences for the quality of life being experienced by the patient. You will often see reference to the QALY in UK healthcare decision-making because it is the preferred outcome measure of NICE (the National Institute for Health and Clinical Excellence).

Capturing costs and benefits

So, once we have identified and quantified our health outcomes, our next task is to consider the cost of the treatment against these benefits.

'Cost is just the price, isn't it?'

Well, as I am sure you're learning, from a health economist's perspective, there's a little bit more to it than that. We must make a clear distinction between the 'financial' and 'economic' concepts of cost.

Financial costs do clearly mean the price of goods or services.

Economic costs, however, try to capture the hidden costs, i.e. those impacts which don't always have a nice neat price tag on them. So, the time spent by patients sitting in a hospital waiting room, or indeed the time spent by their families caring for them at home don't have a price tag, but clearly represent real costs to patients and carers. In *Example 2.1*, suppose Wonderleve had to be delivered by a hospital injection, whereas Average-aid was a tablet to be taken at home – this difference has an impact on both the patient's time and potential discomfort, but doesn't have a particular easily defined financial cost.

So when thinking about economic costs, we have to think of the broader impact of a decision; as you will see, there is more to this than simply looking at the financial costs of our decision.

Opportunity cost

If we spend our budget on Wonderleve for migraine then there would no longer be a budget for Average-aid. The resources have been used, so are now unavailable for use in developing other services, or for duplicating care options. This means that any benefits arising from the use of Average-aid have to be forgone. This is the '**opportunity cost**' of our decision. In reality, we all know this to be true; we all know this from managing our personal finances, or at least trying to..! If the resources at my disposal would allow me to buy either a new suit or a new laptop, in a very real sense, the true opportunity cost of buying the suit is the forgone benefit of using the laptop.

Now I admit, it is really hard to try to measure all the forgone benefits in reality, but opportunity cost does give us a really useful guide in thinking through decisions to the very end, as it clearly shows the explicit trade-offs that have to be made when allocating resources in the health services.

Cost-effectiveness

Health economics (more specifically, health economic evaluation) is structured around a beautiful theoretical concept. One that we all feel we understand, and often talk about without fully considering. That concept is cost-effectiveness, more usually talked about as 'value for money' day to day.

Ultimately, the concept of cost-effectiveness suggests that we want to get the most we can for the least cost. Or put another way, we want to achieve a certain outcome or objective, at the least cost. So, we may want to maximize the health of our population by using our limited resources fully. But how can we identify the 'optimum' way to do this? Well, this is where the tools of economic evaluation are used to try to understand this. Economists will always aim to select the most cost-effective option from the wide range of healthcare alternatives, and equally they would also want to select the more efficient use of resources to achieve this.

Efficiency

Efficiency is simply a measure of how well resources are being used to deliver a particular outcome. That may be an oversimplification as efficiency does have different aspects wrapped within it, but broadly speaking this is correct. You may have heard of the concept of **allocative efficiency**. This is a measure of how well resources are given to the groups or individuals (or patients) who have the highest capacity to benefit from them.

Let's talk this one through a bit. Let's think about our migraine medication Wonderleve again. Imagine we had two groups of patients: those who were at a high risk of migraine, and those with a low risk of migraine. If Wonderleve was demonstrably better at treating high-risk patients than Average-aid, then it's safe to say that the benefits of giving high-risk patients Wonderleve are greater than they would be if Wonderleve were prescribed to low-risk patients.

Giving the high-risk patients Wonderleve is therefore allocatively efficient. If we know this, then we should prioritize giving Wonderleve to the high-risk group, which would of course lead to a greater level of health for the population than if Wonderleve were prescribed to anyone suffering with a migraine.

You may also have heard of **technical efficiency**; this is slightly more complex. Technical efficiency can measure either how well resources are combined to achieve a maximum outcome, or conversely it can measure the minimum amounts of resources that need to be used to achieve a given outcome. We could use technical efficiency to find the least expensive way to effectively treat an ear infection, for example. If we are prescribing unnecessary drugs, or if we are prescribing too many drugs for too long, or perhaps if we are prescribing expensive branded drugs when a cheaper generic version is available and works just as well, then we may be guilty of technical inefficiency.

Perspective

When thinking about economic evaluations, we really do need to think about whose point of view is important to inform that decision. There are a few viewpoints to choose from here; none of these perspectives are 'incorrect', some perspectives are simply more appropriate at times than others. As always, this depends on the decision which is being informed.

One economic analysis could take the perspective of the health service; in this instance only the direct costs would be considered. Equally the analysis could be performed from a societal viewpoint, and here we would seek to include a measure of the indirect costs, perhaps thinking about including productivity losses arising from not attending work. Neither is 'wrong'; they are simply different approaches used to inform a difficult decision.

Generally, health economists tend to prefer the **societal perspective**, as it greatly reduces the risk that any important costs might be missed out from the analysis, as it is the broadest perspective to take. Some costs may be overlooked using other perspectives as these costs may not directly affect the health service, or healthcare provider. We must bear in mind, though, that a healthcare manager who is working with a very limited budget is very much inclined (and often right) to think solely about the costs that have a direct and clear impact on their own budget.

Using a societal perspective does, however, have the advantage of including impacts directly felt by the patient. Consider if Wonderleve was a once a day tablet formulation, replacing the 'three times a day after meals' tablet formulation of Average-aid. Wonderleve would arguably provide a benefit to the patient, perhaps through greater ease of use, with fewer tablets to carry around with them, and with less opportunity to forget to take the tablet. These costs and benefits, which affect the patients directly, could be missed out of an analysis undertaken from a health service perspective. However, these considerations could be thought of as a key part of an economic analysis. The different formulations could improve patient compliance with the therapy, and could mean greater disease control for the patient. This would hopefully lead to an improvement in the health of the patient, and a reduction in the costs borne by society as a result of poorly-controlled migraines. This example gives a brief demonstration of how economic analyses should ideally take the widest possible perspective. By doing so, these analyses maximize their value to decision-makers and could become an invaluable part of healthcare decision-making.

Economic evaluation

Economic evaluation, as we've discussed, does provide a straightforward, systematic and objective framework which allows economists to clearly compare the costs of a new healthcare treatment against the benefits the new treatment may bring. This information can be invaluable and enable decision-makers to come to a more robust conclusion. The comparison of costs and benefits is the common structure on which all economic evaluations are based. All involve a measurement of the inputs ('costs') and a comparison against the health outcomes ('benefits') which the intervention hopes to deliver.

This book considers three main methods of economic evaluation–the three that are most commonly used in healthcare economics. Each method approaches the cost side of the equation in the same rigorous way; this is because costs are often easiest to quantify. It's cost accounting really. However, there is variation in how the health outcomes generated are measured, because capturing these can be quite tricky! We will revisit these economic evaluation types later in the book, but here's a taster.

Cost minimization analysis (Chapter 3)

Cost minimization analysis simply tries to find the least-cost approach from all the alternatives.

This type of approach has to be restricted to situations in which the health outcomes of each alternative have been proven to be identical –this doesn't happen very often, so, in the majority of circumstances, we can't or shouldn't use a cost minimization analysis.

There are some cases, however, where we can use the cost minimization approach. The classic example is if we are thinking of substituting a generic drug for a brand name drug. Imagine we had Wonderleve and generic wonderleve available and that the generic version was a tenth of the cost of the branded Wonderleve. Here we could easily swap the branded drug for the generic drug and achieve the same health outcomes at a far lower cost.

This technique is perceived as being the easiest to apply, and when done badly, it is. To justify the use of this technique, you require hard proof that the health outcomes generated by each drug are clinically equivalent.

What do we mean by 'clinically equivalent'? Well, we will revisit this later in the book but it is wrong to simply assume that interventions for the same condition will give exactly the same outcomes just because they treat the same condition.

Do you think a once a day treatment will give the same outcomes as a twice a day treatment? Does aspirin give the same health outcomes as paracetamol? Can you be sure? Really? You have to tread very carefully before conducting or believing a cost minimization analysis.

Cost-effectiveness analysis (Chapter 4)

This form of analysis is more robust and is often used in health economics. It is a favourite method of evaluation when comparing competing drug treatments. Cost-effectiveness analysis compares the financial costs against health outcomes which are measured as simple health effects. These could be years of life saved, or even something like migraine attacks avoided.

This approach does have some drawbacks; cost-effectiveness analysis is often unable to make comparisons between different treatments which may have slightly different benefits; perhaps one treatment reduces the *number* of migraine attacks, while the other reduces the *severity* of the attacks. But we'll review this important aspect in more detail later in the book.

Cost utility analysis (Chapter 9)

The great advantage of cost utility analysis compared to cost minimization and cost-effectiveness analyses is that it can, in theory at least, draw some comparisons between different treatments in greatly differing areas of healthcare. This is possible because we are converting all the health outcomes achieved into the same unit, the QALY or quality-adjusted life year.

To be honest though, this really isn't easy. QALYs are subject to much debate, as their use can draw a lot of criticisms. On occasion QALYs have been used when they may not have been fully appropriate (in mental health, for example). QALYs will be fully explored in this book, as they really are being used more and more in health economic analysis.

BOX 2.1 WATCH OUT FOR COST BENEFIT ANALYSIS!

Cost benefit analysis –the layman's favourite term.

Whenever you see an economist, or an economic analysis presented in the media, the chances are they will be talking about performing a 'cost benefit analysis' of some description. Now in reality, this won't strictly be true. The media tend to simplify a lot of what economists get up to (and with good reason, if we're honest) but this can lead to some confusion as to what has actually been conducted by the economist.

A cost benefit analysis in health economics is a very specific type of economic analysis where the health outcome for the patient is measured in *cash terms*. Can you see the difficulty with this already? We tend not to be very good at converting our state of health into cash equivalents. How much do we value a day without a migraine? Would £20 cover it? £50? If I gave you £100, would you be happy to have a migraine attack? How much money would you need to compensate you for suffering with migraine?

Needless to say, this approach is not widely used within health economics.

Checking the data and dealing with uncertainty

Economics is uncertain because life is. The world of financial economics has done a great job recently of showing everyone just how uncertain economics can be.

Economics is a behavioural science and is therefore drenched in uncertainty. There's uncertainty around what the exact value of the true cost of treatment might be. There's uncertainty around the true benefit the treatment will deliver to patients in the real world. Almost every variable you can think of will have some degree of uncertainty to it, because nothing is absolutely certain (apart from death and taxes, right?)

To help minimize these uncertainties, economists have to be consistent and accurate in our use of the scientific evidence which underpins our analyses. This is largely done through the use of **evidence-based medicine** techniques. We really do have to be careful to make sure we use a balanced, accurate and impartial summary of all the evidence available to predict treatment outcomes. In an ideal world, these data would come from a full **systematic review**, or perhaps from a well-conducted **meta-analysis**, which would be used to inform our estimate of the treatment benefits. We'll think about these data sources more, later in the book.

Inevitably though, there will be areas where the clinical evidence is either very limited or in some cases just not there. On these occasions it becomes necessary to make some assumptions. It's what economists are famous for, making assumptions, isn't it?

So, to make sure we are confident in our assumptions, health economic analyses must include a **sensitivity analysis** which clearly shows how robust the analysis is. If we can vary our assumptions quite a lot, and not change the outcome of our model, then we can say that the model is robust. If, however, there are changes in the results, and sometimes these variations can change the final outcome and turn the analysis completely on its head, then the economic analysis is not robust. At all. This is a very important element to look for in an economic evaluation, so we will discuss this topic later in more detail.

Final thoughts

Health economics is an exceptionally valuable tool to help us to make good healthcare decisions. It's a way of thinking, really, enabling informed discussions around these issues, which I hope I have introduced here.

Health economic evaluation really can help to structure the decision-making process which inevitably goes alongside every treatment choice, and hopefully a well-conducted analysis can improve the choices made. Being able to understand the processes a health economist goes through when identifying the alternative treatment options, and understanding how they build their models really can help you to understand the literature, and help you understand why certain treatments are chosen, and others rejected.

We've covered a lot in this chapter, but hopefully you are now thinking a little bit like an economist. The rest of the book will guide you through all the key elements of any health economic evaluation and help you to understand a health economic analysis without having becoming an economist yourself, fun though that is..!

3 Cost minimization analysis

...If it's cheap it must be good, right?

What is it?

Cost minimization analysis measures and compares the input costs of competing alternative treatments, assuming the outcomes to be absolutely equivalent. So, the only variable of interest in the analysis is the cost of the treatments.

Introduction

When we think of two treatments which have exactly the same outcome, it is natural to think of the straightforward comparison of branded drugs with their generic equivalents. Generic drugs are chemical equivalents of a branded drug. For a generic medication to be approved for clinical use, the manufacturer must clearly show the authorities (for example, the Food and Drug Administration – the FDA – in the USA) that their product is completely equivalent to the branded medication in terms of pharmaceutical properties.

So, when we want to compare drugs which are chemically identical, using the same doses, and it is obvious that the alternatives have exactly the same pharmaceutical properties as each other, then the cost of the medication is the key comparison, because all the other healthcare outcomes should be the same.

Cost minimization analysis is important, and can be useful, but you do have to be 100% sure that this approach really does make sense for the decision being thought about, and that it does not represent an oversimplification of the decision you are considering.

What sort of questions should this be used to address?

'My practice is considering swapping from a branded to a generic diuretic – is cost minimization analysis appropriate to check if this will really save the practice money?'

How important is this concept? ✪✪✪✪✪

For some people obtaining 'value for money' means that they want to spend the least amount of money they can, to buy what it is they want to buy. This is clearly one approach we could adopt to try to maximize the impact of a given budget, and this approach definitely has its place in healthcare decision-making.

With that said, we really have to be careful to ensure that when we are using this approach to assess resource allocation, it really is the most appropriate approach that we could take. There is a lot to consider, but initially we should think about the bigger context of the comparison being made. For example:

- Could there be unintended consequences associated with treatment (which may also incur a range of additional costs) which are not reflected in the purchase price being asked? If one treatment is a once a day formulation, and the other is a three times a day formulation, then there is a difference in the time costs for the patient. If so, then cost minimization may not appropriate.

- Could there be more side-effects with one treatment than with the other? If there are more side-effects, these might need treatment, and that would incur a cost. Sometimes the cost of treating the side-effects can be greater than the difference in price between the treatments under consideration. Equally, side-effects can seriously impact the health outcome of a patient, which would also rule out a cost minimization approach.

These are not the only dimensions to consider, but they can be a good starting point to guide your assessment of the approach undertaken.

How easy is this idea to understand?

Conceptually, this type of analysis is very straightforward. At its most basic, cost minimization analysis can be summarized quite simply: if you have two different options to choose from, and if both options would generate *exactly the same outcomes*, then quite naturally you should choose the cheapest. This is a fairly intuitive type of analysis.

When is this type of analysis used?

I have to be very clear here: cost minimization analysis should only be used when you are *absolutely certain* that there is total equivalence between the outcomes associated with the options you are choosing between. Ideally, this assumption of equivalence should be supported by good quality clinical evidence, showing clearly that the measured outcomes of interest are indeed equivalent. If this isn't possible, then this type of analysis really shouldn't be used, as there could be other unexpected consequences associated with your decision which may have a cost, and this cost could affect the overall adoption decision. There is a real risk of the incorrect decision being made if the 'hidden' costs outweigh the expected savings identified in the original analysis.

> ## EXAMPLE 3.1 COST MINIMIZATION ANALYSIS
>
> Let us imagine that you have to choose between two pharmaceutical treatments. One is a branded once a day drug which costs £10, and the other is a clinically proven, chemically equivalent once a day generic drug which costs £2. Which should you choose?
>
> Well, given that these drugs have been proven to be chemically equivalent, and are both once a day preparations, then we can be confident that both drugs would give *exactly the same outcomes*. In this example, the generic drug would be better value for money as it can be used to treat 5 patients for the same price as treating one person with the branded drug.

If there is any doubt about equivalence in outcomes between the two alternatives being considered, then a **cost-effectiveness analysis** should be conducted to inform the allocation decision (see *Chapter 4*).

It is important to make this distinction. In my experience in healthcare, the most cost-effective option is very rarely the same as the least cost option, but it is easy and quite natural to fall into this way of thinking. It is easy to assume that two drugs with the same indication must have the same outcomes, so clearly you must choose the cheapest? But, without conducting a cost-effectiveness analysis to test your assumptions, you will be making a decision based upon assumptions which may or may not be true. This can be very costly in the long run. Not only can side-effects be different, but efficacy rates can vary, and the burden on the patient can be quite different if, for example, one drug is an oral tablet and the other is a three times a day injection. These differences will affect your analysis and may lead to a different adoption decision when correctly taken into consideration.

What do the results of a cost minimization analysis mean?

Just to make the point again (sorry but it is important!), if the outcomes between two competing clinical options have genuinely been demonstrated to be equivalent, in high quality published clinical data, then the cheaper option should be the preferred option. This is simply because you would be buying the same 'amount' of health for the least cost. Or, to put it another way, you are buying the most health for your population that you can for your given budget.

Understanding the real outcomes of the treatments is crucial here. Are the outcomes going to be exactly the same regardless of which treatment is chosen? Are you really going to be buying exactly the same outcome as the alternative? If so, then there are clearly some occasions where this type of analysis does make sense, and in these cases, it would be wholly appropriate to choose the cheapest option available, but these situations are very few and far between.

What to watch out for...

Clearly, the big assumption with this kind of analysis is that of equivalence of outcomes:

- If you are not sure that the outcomes are going to be *exactly* the same, then this isn't the appropriate analysis to use

- If in doubt, try to check back to the original clinical data.

Often, the justification for the assumption of equivalence can be open to interpretation, or sometimes there is simply a misinterpretation of the clinical data being presented. If you are in any doubt about the true equivalence of the options being assessed (and remember that the outcomes have to be *identical in every way*), then it is always a good idea to refer back to the clinical source data. Remember, any economic evaluation really is only as good as the quality of the medical evidence supporting it.

4 Cost-effectiveness analysis

The most cost-effective option? Well, that all depends...

What is it?

Cost-effectiveness analysis is used to accurately measure and compare the costs and benefits of various treatments. This enables us to calculate the relative efficiency of the treatments so that the healthcare budget can be allocated most appropriately.

More formally, cost-effectiveness analysis compares the cost of an intervention to its effectiveness as measured in natural health outcomes.

Introduction

Cost-effectiveness analysis helps identify ways to redirect resources to achieve more. It shows the benefits associated with allocating resources from ineffective to effective interventions, and also the benefit of allocating resources from less to more cost-effective interventions.

> ### EXAMPLE 4.1 COST-EFFECTIVENESS ANALYSIS
>
> Imagine a country is spending US$20 billion on healthcare every year and is saving 592 000 lives.
>
> A cost-effectiveness analysis could investigate the many different ways of allocating these healthcare funds, and may well find that the number of lives saved could be doubled if the same $20 billion were reallocated to much more cost-effective interventions. It could be that US$20 billion spent purely on lung cancer treatment is not as effective, in terms of lives saved, as spending the same amount on a meningitis vaccination programme.

How important is this concept?   ✪ ✪ ✪ ✪ ✪

Cost-effectiveness analysis is probably **the** most important concept in the field of health economic evaluation. This analysis is the foundation for many of the evaluation approaches discussed within this book.

Cost-effectiveness analyses are used when we want to examine and evaluate the costs associated with, and health effects of, a specific healthcare treatment or strategy. We then go on to assess the extent to which this new treatment can be thought of as providing good 'value for money' when compared with a different treatment.

Cost-effectiveness analyses are being used to justify healthcare decisions more and more, in many different countries and settings around the globe. You will always be at an advantage if you can understand the basic concepts which drive a cost-effectiveness analysis.

How easy is this to understand?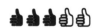

Cost-effectiveness analyses can often be relatively straightforward, or they can be very complex indeed, depending upon the options which are being evaluated. However, this approach still comes down to comparing the total cost of an intervention against the total benefits associated with that intervention, and then comparing this against the current treatment paradigm, or any other alternatives available.

A cost-effectiveness analysis is designed purely to compare the costs and health effects of an intervention (be it pharmaceutical, technological, or surgical), with another intervention. This is often a comparison against the current standard of care.

Cost-effectiveness analysis formally assesses the degree to which an intervention can be thought of as providing 'value for money' – this can be applied to society as a whole, an organization or hospital – in comparison to an alternative.

The most difficult part of a cost-effectiveness analysis is often how the benefits, specifically health benefits, are captured and measured.

When is this type of analysis used?

Cost-effectiveness analyses are probably the most commonly used in health economic evaluation, because they are often used to inform and guide healthcare decision-makers who have the difficult job of determining where to allocate limited healthcare resources.

What do the results of a cost-effectiveness analysis mean?

The big difference between a cost-effectiveness analysis and a cost minimization analysis (see *Chapter 3*), is that in a cost-effectiveness analysis we acknowledge that different treatments tend to have different outcomes for patients as well as different cost profiles.

A cost-effectiveness analysis captures the differences in health outcomes in natural units; that is, the differences between the treatments are presented in terms which make sense for the disease or condition being reviewed, for example:

- life years gained are often used if the treatments offer an improvement in survival

- event-free days can be used if the treatment can reduce the frequency of episodes of illness

- pain-free days will be used if the treatments can reduce the pain a patient is experiencing.

Cost-effectiveness ratio

Because a cost-effectiveness analysis compares different treatments and different outcomes, the results are often reported as a **cost-effectiveness ratio (CER)**. This enables us to quickly make comparisons between the various treatment options.

BOX 4.1 COST-EFFECTIVENESS RATIOS

CER = Costs of new intervention/Health effects generated (e.g. life years gained)

This formula remains the same, regardless of how the health effects generated are measured, as long as they are measured using natural units (such as life years gained, or event-free days).

For example:

New treatment costs £300 and gives 20 event-free days

CER = £300/20 event-free days = £15 per event-free day

Incremental cost-effectiveness ratio

In real life, we often have to make choices between different treatments or technologies which are **mutually exclusive**; that is, we can only adopt one of them, and when we adopt it, we forgo the other alternative.

When we choose to treat a patient with a particular treatment, this is normally in place of a different treatment, so the choice is a mutually exclusive one. In this case, the key questions are:

- *'What are the additional benefits we are gaining from the new treatment?'*

- *'What are the additional costs (if any) associated with the new treatment?'*

Here, we are conducting an **incremental cost-effectiveness** analysis (these incremental analyses are how we address most of our healthcare decisions). *How much more* would treatment X cost over treatment Y? *How much more* benefit does treatment X deliver over treatment Y?

This analysis leads us to generate an **incremental cost-effectiveness ratio (ICER)**:

EXAMPLE 4.2 INCREMENTAL COST-EFFECTIVENESS RATIO

ICER = Difference in cost between treatments/difference in health effects between treatments

So, let's work this through. Say treatment A costs £50 000 and B costs £100 000, and treatment A adds 5 life years and treatment B adds 7.2 life years.

ICER = Difference in cost between treatments/difference in health effects between treatments

ICER = £50 000/2.2

ICER = £22 727 per life year gained

We are often presented at the end of a cost-effectiveness analysis with an ICER. In our example above, the ICER generated is £22 727 per life year gained. But is this good value for money?

The 'threshold' of acceptability for value for money will vary from country to country and is generally set by the decision-maker. In England and Wales, there is a very loose rule of thumb that under £30 000 per life year gained is acceptable. The National Institute of Health and Clinical Excellence (NICE) uses a cost utility analysis approach (see *Chapter 8*) but an implicit threshold is understood to be around the £30 000 per quality-adjusted life year (we'll talk a lot more about the QALY in *Chapter 7*).

Cost-effectiveness plane

Once we have the results of our cost-effectiveness analyses, it is common practice to place these on what is commonly referred to as the **cost-effectiveness plane** (see *Figure 4.1*).

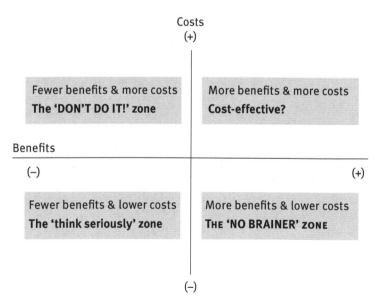

FIGURE 4.1 The cost-effectiveness plane

Each quadrant of the cost-effectiveness plane has a different implication for the policy adoption decision.

- If the ICER falls in the 'no brainer' quadrant, with lower costs and positive effects, then the intervention would be more effective (i.e. may have better survival) and less costly than the alternative. Interventions falling in this quadrant are always considered cost-effective, for obvious reasons.

- If the ICER falls in the 'don't do it!' quadrant, with higher costs and negative effects, then the new technology would be more costly and less effective than the current option (i.e. the new technology is 'dominated' by the standard). Interventions falling in this quadrant are never, ever, considered cost-effective!

- If the ICER falls in the 'cost-effective?' quadrant, with higher costs and positive effects, or in the 'think seriously' quadrant, with lower costs and negative effects. In both of these, the trade-offs between costs and effects would need to be considered. These two quadrants represent the situation where the new technology **may** be cost-effective when compared to the standard treatment, but this is all dependent upon the value at which the ICER is generally considered good value for money.

You need to be careful here. When reviewing a cost-effectiveness analysis think carefully about the decision being made. If the decision is between two competing treatments and the proposal is only to adopt one (if we can only afford to adopt one, for example), then the treatments under consideration are mutually exclusive options. In this case you need to look for the use of incremental cost-effectiveness ratios in the analysis and these ICERs will show the incremental benefit of one option over the other.

Non-mutually exclusive decisions

Sometimes there will be non-mutually exclusive decisions which have to be made. That is, there may be the opportunity to fund treatment A for asthma, and treatment B for blepharitis, and treatment C for chronic fatigue. All could be done. But what if we only had a limited budget? Which should we fund first? Here we use **average cost-effectiveness** ratios. To calculate this you simply divide the cost of providing the treatment by the benefit the treatment gives. Let's work through an example:

Treatment	Event-free days	Net cost
A	50	£1000
B	3	£ 300
C	40	£1200

The average cost-effectiveness = net cost/net health benefit = £/ event-free days.

The average cost-effectiveness of treatment A = net cost/net health benefit = £1000/50 event-free days= £20/event-free day.

Using the same logic, the average cost-effectiveness for intervention B is £100/event-free day and the average cost-effectiveness for intervention C is £30/event-free day.

If the health authority only has £2500 to spend on these health interventions, which one of these health interventions should they fund first?

Well, let's put them in order of average cost-effectiveness and have a look:

Treatment	Event-free days	Net cost	Average CE (£/event-free day)
A	50	£1000	£ 20/event-free day
C	40	£1200	£ 30/event-free day
B	3	£ 300	£100/event-free day

Treatment A should be paid for first because it has the best (lowest) cost-effectiveness ratio compared to the other interventions (i.e. £20/EFD vs. £30/EFD or £100/EFD). This would be the most efficient way to spend this money rather than by starting funding one of the other interventions which has a higher average cost-effectiveness ratio. So, what would come next if the health authority still had money left over? Well, C would be the next best treatment to cover, followed by B if there was still any money left.

Perspective

The **perspective** of the analysis is also very important. Whether or not an intervention is considered to be cost-effective will depend upon the perspective of the analysis you take. A **societal perspective** is the broadest perspective for the analysis that you can take, and includes all the possible costs and benefits which may arise as a result of the intervention used.

However, other perspectives are often used: NICE in England and Wales uses the perspective of the NHS in England and Wales. This means that any costs which are incurred by a patient are not included in the analysis. So, if a patient incurs transportation costs, such as a bus fare, to attend a clinic in the hospital, then these costs are not included in the analysis because they do not impact the NHS and so fall outside of the 'NHS perspective'.

Additionally, if two treatments under comparison had different treatment schedules, say a once a week hospital infusion versus a once a day hospital infusion, then the additional costs of nurse time and ward time would be included from the 'NHS perspective', but the additional time costs for the patient and their additional transportation costs would not. The perspective of the study can and does alter the conclusions of analysis.

Cost-effectiveness analyses and budgets

The cost-effectiveness ratios reported should always be considered against the available budget, to help us pick the most cost-effective strategies appropriate for our situation. Something can be very cost-effective indeed but still be too expensive to adopt.

EXAMPLE 4.3 COST-EFFECTIVE DOES NOT MEAN CHEAP!

I know that I would enjoy owning and driving a classic Ferrari very much indeed. I know that they hold their value very well. So, in cost-effectiveness terms, a Ferrari can be thought of as a cost-effective option and this could be a perfect justification for the acquisition of a fabulous car, as I'm sure you'll agree.

The only problem is that regardless of how cost-effective an option the classic Ferrari is, no matter how great the value for money it offers, I simply can't afford to buy one! I am limited by my budget.

The same thing can and does happen in healthcare. Cataract surgery has been shown to be a very cost-effective procedure. However, many health authorities in the UK are restricting access to this treatment as the total volume of procedures required means they simply cannot afford to treat everyone immediately. They are thus denying cost-effective care to patients because of budgetary constraints.

What to watch out for...

- How good are the clinical data supporting the analysis?

- Has a sensitivity analysis been conducted?

- From whose perspective has the analysis been done?

All cost-effectiveness analyses are based upon clinical data. So we need to be sure that the clinical data used are appropriate and accurate. The clinical data themselves contain a margin for error, in terms of **confidence intervals** around the outcomes reported. As such, all cost-effectiveness analyses should also allow margins of error.

Cost-effectiveness analysis is a far from precise science, and we know that there is often a large degree of uncertainty associated with the findings of any economic analysis. So, we must make an allowance for these uncertainties, both in the inputs and the assumptions we make within the analysis. This process of allowing for the uncertainties within the approach is called **sensitivity analysis** (see *Chapter 8*) and should always be routinely included. Remember, cost-effectiveness data are just another piece of information helping a decision-maker to make their choice. The quality of a cost-effectiveness analysis is very much related to the quality of the clinical data used to inform it. A sensitivity analysis allows us to check to see how much a change in the parameters used affects the final decision.

We also need to consider the perspective of the analysis. We may need to consider the requirements of the government, national and local health service providers and the patients. All of these will have different requirements and needs. Patients are interested in factors which directly affect them, such as time and travel costs. The NHS manager is not really interested in costs which do not fall within his or her budget, so may only consider the purchase cost of the drug and the staff time required to administer the treatment.

In conclusion, you should always take care when reading cost-effectiveness studies to make sure that all the assumptions the author used are clear, and that the context and perspective of the study are very clear too. You should also check to see if the authors have conducted a sensitivity analysis and then review the final cost-effectiveness ratio and think about how that compares to the 'threshold' in your country. Remember, it sounds complex but ultimately we are simply comparing the costs against the benefits and seeing if we think that the benefits outweigh the costs!

5 Quality of life

Why health economic analysis is different...

What is it?

Quality of life (QoL) is a term which is used to measure or quantify the general wellbeing of individuals and, in some cases, of societies and countries.

You will find that this term is used in a wide range of contexts within healthcare. Quality of life generally focuses on physical and mental health, recreation and leisure time, and social belonging.

Remember not to confuse this with standard of living, which is based primarily on income.

Introduction

Quality of life can be thought of in many ways by many different people, making its measurement problematic: if we can't measure it well, then putting a quality of life questionnaire into a clinical trial can also be difficult.

Illnesses, diseases and ailments undoubtedly have an impact on a patient's quality of life; any treatment given could also affect a patient's mood; and there could also be side-effects which may limit their ability to see family and friends. If the side-effects stop them being able to work, their economic wellbeing could also be affected.

So, any definition of quality of life should try to be as all-encompassing as possible, to truly capture the patient's experience, as well as allowing health professionals to see which areas of a patient's life are affected, and in which way, by any given treatment. This would then allow a comparison of different treatments for the same condition, not only in terms of efficacy, but also in terms of impact on a patient's quality of life.

What sort of questions should this be used to address?

'I have two treatment options for my patient:

- one resolves symptoms quickly but may cause temporary hair loss

- the other option is a month-long treatment which also resolves the symptoms but only at the end of the treatment; this treatment doesn't cause hair loss, but the symptoms of the disease remain for longer

Which treatment will have the least impact on my patient's quality of life?'

A well-developed quality of life questionnaire would allow a clinical trial comparing these treatments to be able to answer this question and to help inform us which treatment has the least impact on a patient's quality of life.

How important is this concept? ✪✪✪✪✪

We all use the term 'quality of life' in our everyday lives. Many people talk about improving their quality of life, perhaps wishing for a better quality of life or speculating on whether or not the quality of life is better in Switzerland than in London (or maybe even the other way around!). People use the term 'quality of life' in a multitude of different ways, often capturing many different concepts within it (cost of living, disposable income, free time). In health economic evaluation, we have to be very careful how we define 'quality of life' as we clearly want to be able to establish whether or not a technology or intervention can improve a person's quality of life, specifically their **health-related quality of life (HRQoL)**. But we also want to be able to do this consistently across many different treatments, technologies or interventions, in many different settings.

So, if quality of life can be defined in many different ways, this can clearly make its measurement and incorporation into clinical trials very difficult. This in turn means that we have to be careful when thinking about it from a health economic perspective. Specifically in health economics we talk about health-related quality of life, as we want to examine the impact a person's health has on quality of life, rather than other factors such as income or environment. Ultimately the person's health will hopefully be improved by the technology or treatment we are assessing.

How easy is this idea to understand?
👍👍👍👍👍

This idea is very natural for us to take on. We all know that we feel terrible when we are ill, and feel much better when we are well. Equally, we know that different types of illnesses affect us in different ways. A broken leg would clearly affect our physical abilities but probably wouldn't impair our ability to do a crossword. Equally, a broken leg would only slightly affect my ability to do my work, whereas if I was a premiership footballer playing for Manchester United…

With these differences in mind we can explore the key components of health-related quality of life assessment – these are sometimes called the core domains of a multidimensional HRQoL questionnaire:

- physical
- functional
- psychological/emotional
- social/occupational

Ideally each of these domains should be able to be assessed independently of the others, so we can establish the true impact of an intervention, and where it has the most impact on a patient's health-related quality of life.

When is health-related quality of life (HRQoL) used?

The primary purpose of any treatment is to improve the quality of life of the patient, hopefully by successfully treating and curing the condition they are suffering from. But this is not always possible and so some treatments are designed to ameliorate the worst symptoms of a disease for as long as possible. Also, some treatments may have unavoidable side-effects which, whilst treating the underlying condition, can greatly detract from a patient's quality of life. In extreme cases, some patients may choose to not have the treatment as the impact of that treatment on their quality of life is too great for them to bear. This is why HRQoL is such an important factor for health economists to take into consideration.

Sometimes, the improvements in HRQoL can really outweigh any other concerns, even financial, if the improvements are great enough.

Remember though that these improvements do not necessarily have to be in the physical domain; for example, there may be a new treatment developed which shows no improvement in efficacy over the standard treatment. So why would you recommend a change to the new treatment if it offers no improvement in clinical outcome? Well, if the new treatment was a once a day tablet for a chronic condition and was replacing a three times a day injection, then patients quite rightly may express a preference for the oral treatment, since it offers an improvement in the social/occupational domain.

How is health-related quality of life measured?

It is important that we think about how HRQoL is measured scientifically. The way that we assess patient-reported outcomes has become much more sophisticated in recent years. The questionnaires used nowadays are much more robust and all the questionnaires used are tested to ensure that they genuinely do measure changes in HRQoL, i.e. they are valid, responsive to change and reliable.

A generic HRQoL questionnaire is one that has been designed and validated for use with patients suffering from ANY disease or condition. This inevitably means that the questions in a generic questionnaire are less specific and therefore more general, but this 'generalizability' enables us to make comparisons across disease states, as well as making comparisons for different treatments within the same condition.

BOX 5.1 A GENERIC HRQoL QUESTIONNAIRE SHORT FORM 36

I expect that many of you will already have heard of probably the most important and frequently-used generic HRQoL questionnaire, the **short form 36 (SF-36)**. This is a multi-purpose, short-form health questionnaire which is made up of 36 questions and can be used to generate a profile of functional health and wellbeing scores, across eight areas:

- physical function

- role function (work or other daily activities)

- bodily pain

- general health

- vitality

- social functioning

- emotional wellbeing

- mental health.

This questionnaire has been utilized in thousands of general and specific population surveys. The large data sets generated have allowed researchers to make comparisons of the relative burden of diseases, and enabled a clear differentiation of the health benefits or harms of many different treatments. An important aspect about the SF-36 is that the burden on the patient is not that great: the questions are straightforward and there are not that many of them. But, should some people consider 36 questions to be too many, there is also an even shorter validated version, the SF-12, available and this asks, unsurprisingly, just 12 questions.

Both these HRQoL instruments have been reliably translated into many languages and have been used successfully around the world.

In addition to generic questionnaires there are also **disease-specific** questionnaires. Disease-specific questionnaires ask questions which are specific to the disease, so a cancer questionnaire such as the EORTC QLQ-C30 would ask the patient only to report outcomes which are specific to cancer. These answers would then NOT be comparable against someone with Alzheimer's disease or asthma, because the instrument is only **validated** for use with cancer patients.

What to watch out for...

It is important to note that if quality of life or patient-reported outcome data have been collected within a study, it is vital that these data have been collected using a validated and well-recognized instrument. Always check whether:

- a validated HRQoL instrument for the disease has been used

- there are any obvious domains being overlooked: mental health impact?, impact on social interactions?

In some cases an instrument may have been developed specifically for the study, and if this is the case it is still important to check that the instrument has been validated for the population under investigation, so that you can be confident in the outcomes reported.

Patient-reported outcomes and HRQoL are becoming increasingly important factors to consider in decision-making and in clinical evidence generation. There are now a number of excellent instruments widely available and there is an increasing evidence base supporting their use.

HRQoL is a key indicator of the positive (and negative) impact of a treatment on a disease and is becoming more accepted in use alongside some of the more traditional objective measures such as symptom-free days, and patient-reported outcomes really do complement these assessments. Just remember to check that the instrument used is appropriate for the study being undertaken!

6 Health utilities

How do you value being healthy..?

What are they?

Health utilities are a tool to help us find out the values patients and society place on certain health outcomes, because they can be complex and sometimes surprising. Utilities are an important tool in health economics as they allow a consistent comparison of outcomes across diseases, populations and programmes.

A utility score is not a monetary value; it is a measure of preference for a particular health-related quality of life.

Introduction

When health economists talk about quality of life, they often talk about utilities in the same breath. Utilities are not the same as health-related quality of life (which is discussed in *Chapter 5*), but they are related.

Health utilities can be applied to individuals, clinical groups, and even general populations. Health utility scores facilitate the measurement and interpretation of results collected in different studies undertaken in different conditions.

In the analysis of health outcomes, a health utility score is simply a number between 0 and 1 which is assigned to a state of health.

- Perfect health has a value of 1.

- Death has a value of 0.

Almost all other health states lie somewhere between, although some health states could be thought of as worse than death (permanent coma, for example) and so a negative utility score is also a possibility.

Utilities are all about an individual's preference for being in a particular health state. Remember though that every individual will have their own individual preferences.

EXAMPLE 6.1 HEALTH STATE PREFERENCES

As an extreme example, imagine that you have to lose one of your five senses. Which one would you be happy to forgo? Your sight? Your hearing? Your sense of smell? Which one would it be? Studies have shown most people would not choose to lose their sight; indeed many people would not choose to lose their hearing either.

So, imagine we asked you which sense would you least like to lose? Which sense do you value the most? The majority of people would choose sight as the sense they value the most, **but not everyone does**. A sound recordist, for example, may value their hearing more than their sight – their utility score for keeping their hearing over their sight would be higher than that of the general population.

How important is this concept? ✪✪✪✪✪

This concept is important simply because you will see many analyses in the published literature which use utilities. Utilities are being applied to more and more diseases and conditions in an attempt to allow comparisons across disease areas which would normally not be thought of as comparable. Utilities can also help to indentify which patients, if any, may have the greatest capacity to benefit from a particular treatment. These data are often used to inform the difficult decisions healthcare providers have to make when faced with a limited healthcare budget. It could be that a decision has to be made between funding a new treatment for glaucoma and developing a keyhole surgery capability for a hospital. A common measure of benefit, such as utilities, enables comparisons of patient benefit across disparate conditions.

How easy is this idea to understand?
👍👍👍👍👍

This can be a tricky subject to understand. However, the idea that two people with the same condition may feel differently about their condition, is relatively intuitive: some people may value being free of pain more than being mobile, while others may prefer to be active and be willing to accept a degree of discomfort in order to be so.

The difficult area is being confident in how these utility values are elicited. We need to be sure that the methods used to elicit the values are valid, just like with HRQoL.

Utilities and the Quality-Adjusted Life Year (QALY) are almost joined at the hip, and as such they have become an increasingly popular outcome measure in pharmaceutical research. Specifically, utilities are often used as the preference weights or quality levels, as part of the QALY, which is covered in more detail in *Chapter 7*.

How do we measure utilities and when are they used?

Measuring health utilities normally involves two main steps.

- The first step is to define exactly which health states we are interested in. What exactly is it we are trying to value?

- Then, quite naturally, the next step is to try to value those health states, and often to place them in a ranking order: 1st, 2nd, 3rd and so on.

This means that utilities are themselves **cardinal values** which reflect an individual's preference for different health outcomes.

There are two different approaches to valuing utilities, and they can generally be thought of as either **direct** or **indirect** valuations.

- Direct valuation (sometimes called direct measurement) tends to be performed for discrete, and occasionally for condition-specific, health states such as visual impairment associated with age-related macular degeneration, or for symptoms associated with diabetic leg ulcers which are specific to that condition.

- Indirect valuation is more complex. It involves applying utility algorithms to questionnaires which are given to the patients. These questionnaires are generally disease-specific, HRQoL instruments. The answers from these questionnaires are then mapped onto a utility algorithm which, generally speaking, converts the disease-specific elements of the questionnaire into the broader generic instrument. The two instruments will not perfectly fit each other, and there will therefore be some 'noise' around the merged data, but this will allow a utility score to be generated. As I say, indirect methods are more complex, but have been used to great effect in medical decision-making.

Both direct and indirect valuations are based around the responses of patients (and the general public) to a series of questions. So the validity of the utility is only ever as good as the quality of the questions being asked. When designing an instrument to directly measure utilities, great care is taken to avoid context effects (see *Box 6.1*) because the way a health state is described can affect the way a patient responds to the question.

BOX 6.1 CONTEXT EFFECTS

Context effects surround us every day. Someone of average height would appear to be tiny when they are playing basketball with much taller professional players, but the same person would look like a giant when supervising a basketball game played by young children.

The context or wording of a question can also affect the answer given by the respondent. Imagine we want to find out how many people in a pub want another drink. We could ask 'Would you like another drink?' to everyone in the pub. This is a perfectly reasonable question to use in this study. However, it is a closed question which can easily be answered with a yes or a no. Once we had asked everyone, we could then tally the results and come to a conclusion.

Imagine if we had instead asked the patrons of the pub 'Would you like a pint or a half?' This question assumes that the person being asked wants another drink. This question has neatly reduced their answer set down to two *positive* outcomes. The context of this question guides the respondent towards a positive answer.

Sales people have been using context effects like this to their advantage for years.

Direct valuation

We have to start by establishing what health states we are interested in. Or, more loosely, which patient outcomes are we interested in? This is important, because if we choose health states which do not match up to patient outcomes, we won't be able to show that there are differences between treatments, even if those differences exist. These health outcomes, or health states (economists often refer to these as 'attributes'), can include mental wellbeing, physical impairments, symptoms and pain. The main thing here is that these attributes are based upon the actual experience of the patient.

Imagine a man suffering from severe arthritis. This disease would affect the patient across multiple attributes. There would be pain, there could also be reduced mobility, and reduced ability to care for himself, and as a result this may also impact his state of mind and mental wellbeing.

So, once we have decided which health states we are interested in for the condition under scrutiny, we then have to value these states. Many different methods can be used but the most common are: **standard gamble**, **time trade-off and rating scales**. I'm not going to go into a lot of detail here (as you don't really need it) but I will give a brief outline of these techniques for your information, as you will see them mentioned in the literature.

Standard gamble

The standard gamble presents individuals with a choice between two alternatives; a health state that is absolutely certain (the condition the patient is currently suffering from), and another health state. This other health state is essentially a gamble between a better outcome (full perfect health) and a much worse outcome (often death).

As *Example 6.2* demonstrates, the standard gamble tries to find at what risk of death you are **indifferent** between staying with the disease and choosing the treatment. At this risk point, you have placed a value on your chronic fatigue. Now we need to find out what that value is as a number.

Put another way, at what probability of perfect health (and also of certain death!) can the patient not choose between the two options? If the respondents are truly indifferent between the chronic fatigue and the gamble with a 0.7 probability of the perfect health outcome (and a 0.3 probability of death), then 0.7 represents the utility score of the chronic fatigue health state. This could then be compared to utility scores from other diseases and conditions generated in the same way.

EXAMPLE 6.2 THE STANDARD GAMBLE

Imagine you suffer from chronic fatigue. Your doctor tells you of a new treatment which completely cures 70% of all patients, and gives them perfect health. The downside of this treatment is that it kills 30% of the patients who take it.

You have the option of continuing with your chronic fatigue, or you could start the treatment – what would you do?

Would you start the treatment if the odds were 60:40, or 80:20, or 90:10? The point at where you honestly cannot decide between starting the treatment and remaining in your current health state is the point we are interested in. This is where you are **indifferent** between staying with the disease and choosing the treatment, and this point of indifference represents your valuation of your current health state.

Time trade-off

This approach asks people to consider relative amounts of time (such as the number of life years) that they would be willing to give up, in order to be able to avoid a guaranteed poorer health state (let's use chronic fatigue again).

EXAMPLE 6.3 TIME TRADE-OFF

Consider a scenario where a patient has the prospect of living for 10 more years but with their chronic fatigue for all of this time; they may be prepared to undergo a treatment which cures their chronic fatigue but which reduces their lifespan by six years, i.e. they will only live for another four years.

If they were to accept the treatment, we would say that the patient is **indifferent** between their current health state and having six years less of life. We therefore have an estimated utility score for the chronic fatigue health state of 0.6 (six years divided by the 10 years).

Rating scale system

This is sometimes called the visual analogue scale approach. The rating scale system is grounded in psychometric theory. It consists of a single line with 'anchors' (a ceiling/floor or left/right walls) which represent the best possible health and the worst possible state; this is normally death but could be some other alternative. *Example 6.4* shows the Oxford Scale used for pain scoring; here the anchors are 'no pain' and 'severe pain'. People are then asked to place each described health state on this line, in such a way that the points they mark on the line reflect their personal perception of the differences between the health states described.

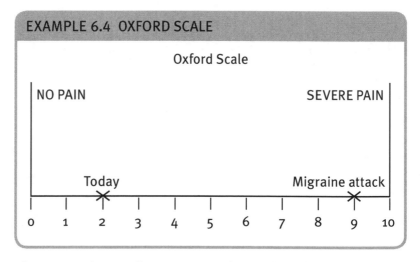

EXAMPLE 6.4 OXFORD SCALE

This approach actually generates values rather than true utilities, because it doesn't involve any element of making a choice, nor does it test an individual's decision-making under uncertainty. But it is often used, and can be considered to be a good proxy to a 'true' utility.

Indirect valuation

Let's quickly think about indirect methods for measuring utilities, through the use of **generic utility instruments** (such as the **Euroqol 5 dimensions** or **EQ-5D**) because you will probably come across this type of approach in the literature as well.

With a generic utility instrument, certain non-disease-specific health states (such as mobility, self care, usual activities, pain/discomfort and anxiety/depression) are identified and placed together for valuation to create a utility score. So we might ask 'How would you value being in pain and being unable to walk around but free from depression?' Answers are then aggregated to generate the utility score for that health state.

A scoring algorithm is then created from the utility scores (using a technique called econometric modelling). This scoring algorithm is then used to calculate utilities for other health states which have not been valued directly.

Patients who are suffering from any health condition can then fill in a relatively simple questionnaire which will define the generic health state they are in, and the scoring algorithm is then applied to the data from this questionnaire to generate the appropriate utility value.

If this all sounds complicated, that's because it is! You don't really need to know much more than the above summary – you should simply check that the generic instrument used is well-validated. Three instruments in common use today are the EQ-5D (Euroqol 5 dimensions), the SF-6D (Short Form 6 dimensions) and the HUI (Health Utilities Index) – these are all high quality instruments and, if one of these has been used, you can be fairly confident of the utilities reported.

Whose preferences are we interested in?

All of the approaches we have described can be asked of patients (or proxies such as parents if required) or of the general public. The main reason for asking the patients themselves is that it is they who have to experience the impact of the disease and any treatments, so we should clearly be considering their preferences.

If we are asking patients, then we can ask them to value a hypothetical health state or their own current health state. Any utilities which we obtain through hypothetical scenarios clearly run the risk of not being the true preferences associated with patients who actually are experiencing those health states. So, if we are asking patients, it will generally be preferable (but often more difficult) to find and then recruit patients with the specific health states that we are interested in.

Why should we ask the preferences of the general public regarding hypothetical health states; where is the value in that? In the UK we have a publicly funded healthcare system. It is society's resources (via taxation) that are paying for the healthcare provision, so it therefore follows that the views of the general population should be taken into account.

Often the perception of the impact of a disease can be greater than the true impact of living with the condition. The expected impact an able-bodied person perceives if we ask them to imagine losing the use of their legs may be greater than the true impact of living in a wheelchair. So, as you can see, whose preference we actually measure is important, because it could well be that utilities we generate vary between different population groups for the same health state.

Broadly speaking, studies suggest that if we ask patients suffering from a disease to generate a utility for a hypothetical health state which is likely to be considered worse than their current health state, they tend to give higher answers than the general public. That is, patients think that the worse hypothetical health state isn't 'as bad' as a healthy person thinks it is. Some health economists think that this effect could be linked to a patient's coping mechanism for living with ill health. If you ask a patient who is fully sighted to value the impact of sight loss, and then ask a person living with sight loss to value their current health state, you will get greatly differing answers. This is often because of **adaptation** (see *Box 6.2*).

BOX 6.2 ADAPTATION

People who are living with sight loss can still enjoy aspects of life that sighted people may think would have been lost to them. Partially sighted or blind people can keep up to date on current affairs by listening to the radio, or using speaking newspapers, when once they may have used the internet. They may enjoy radio plays, where once they watched television. They may have learnt to read Braille, and so can still enjoy literature. An average sighted person may not fully appreciate the impact of these adaptive behaviours when valuing the impact loss of sight may have on their daily lives.

I know we've spent a lot of time on utilities, but it is worth it as they are becoming more and more the currency of health economic evaluation.

What to watch out for...

Utilities can be quite complex to understand, and it is important to remember that the utility scores being considered are only as good as the data gathering on which they are based. Whenever you need to consider treatment options which are based on utility scores you should bear the following three points in mind:

- Have the utilities been generated by a valid method (i.e. EQ-5D, SF-6D or HUI)? Are they just taken from a different study? Is the instrument used recognized for generating utilities, or has an indirect utility generation method (as described above) been used?

- Check to see if the values reported make intuitive sense. Would a utility of 0.9 seem feasible for a comatose patient, when a value of 1 is full perfect health? Equally, would restoring someone's sight following a cataract only provide a 0.001 utility improvement? Do the utility scores presented feel broadly acceptable?

- Are the utility scores generally in line with other, similar studies?

7 The infamous quality-adjusted life year (QALY)

The most misused and misunderstood term in health economics.

What is it?

The quality-adjusted life year (or QALY) is a widely used measure of the burden of a disease, which includes both the *quality*, and the *quantity*, of life lived. The QALY is often used when trying to formally assess the value for money of a healthcare intervention.

The QALY calculated for any treatment is based upon the number of years of life which could be added by the treatment, multiplied by the patient's health utility.

Introduction

The **Quality-Adjusted Life Year**, or QALY, is now one of the most widely used terms within the field of health economics. When you hear researchers, academics and healthcare professionals discuss QALYs, it's likely that you will recognize that they are talking about a health economic evaluation. But in my experience, the QALY is a misused term, and it's not always fully understood by the many people who use the measure.

A QALY is a measure of evaluation which tries to take into account both the quantity of life a person experiences, weighted by the quality of life they experience. Strictly, the quantity of life is weighted by the valuation of the quality of life a person experiences (their utility).

As you will recall, a utility is a number between 0 and 1 that is assigned to a state of health or an outcome. Perfect health has a value of 1. Death has a value of 0. If the extra years gained from a particular treatment are not to be lived in a perfect health state, and almost all are not, then the extra life years achieved are given a value between 0 and 1 to account for this (see *Example 7.1*).

EXAMPLE 7.1 CALCULATING THE QALY

A new treatment offers a patient an additional 10 years of life in perfect health (utility of 1.0). This treatment would therefore generate:

10 yrs x 1.0 = 10 QALYs

An alternative treatment which could only add 5 years with a utility of 0.8 would therefore generate:

5 yrs x 0.8 = 4 QALYs

A third treatment offers 5 years of extra life, but with a utility of 0.4 and therefore generates:

5 yrs x 0.4 = 2 QALYs

We must note though that a simple QALY analysis is concerned only with the resulting benefits in terms of quantity and quality of life of a particular treatment. This approach does not say anything about the costs of these treatments. The analysis of QALYs and costs will be discussed in *Chapter 8* (Cost utility analysis).

How important is this concept?

This concept is important for health economic analyses as it allows comparisons across health states and across diseases.

A QALY allows us to place a different value, or weight, on life lived in different states of health. So, if a person lived for a whole year in a state of complete and perfect health (that is, their health could not be any better at all) then we would weight this year as a 1.

Any time spent in a state of less than perfect health, and let's be honest, that covers pretty much all of us, is valued as less than one. There is a very natural anchor to this scale, death. Death is valued quite rightly as zero, although, as we all know, some health conditions can be considered by many people to be worse than death itself.

How easy is this idea to understand?

QALYs can be difficult. They can feel abstract and not grounded in a patient's true experience.

The real appeal of the QALY is that it can provide comparisons across different disease states (see *Example 7.2*). I always think of trying to compare prices when abroad. Instinctively we all convert the price in the local currency back to our home currency.

> ### EXAMPLE 7.2 QALY COMPARISON ACROSS DISEASES
>
> Can you compare treatment X for acute asthma and treatment Y for chronic arthritis?
>
> Treatment X provides a patient with 10 extra years of life at a utility of 0.5 = 5 QALYs
>
> Treatment Y provides a patient with 5 extra years of life at a utility of 0.4 = 2 QALYs.
>
> By using QALYs, we now have a 'common currency' for the outcomes of these treatments.

As *Example 7.2* shows, the QALY is a 'common currency' for health outcomes, capturing the benefits of a treatment or health intervention both in terms of additional years lived, as well as a measure of the quality of life the person experiences, regardless of the disease. We can therefore compare the outcomes of these treatments directly as they are now measured in the same common currency. The asthma treatment (X) provides more benefit than the arthritis treatment (Y) in this example.

As mentioned earlier, this basic QALY analysis doesn't take the costs of each treatment into consideration. Obviously, if the asthma treatment is cheaper than the arthritis treatment then this is now a simple decision. It becomes more difficult to call when the treatment with the higher QALYs is also more costly. We will examine this more in *Chapter 8*.

Should we always use QALYs?

Health economists agree that the QALY isn't perfect: there are a number of methodological and technical issues with it. However, QALYs are being used more and more in medical decision-making, including their use in informing very serious healthcare resourcing decisions.

The use of the QALY does mean that these difficult choices, between what are essentially competing patient groups with differing conditions and diseases, are made explicit. As a result of this, decision-makers are being made aware of the potential benefits from investment in new and/or alternative technologies. These decisions will always be difficult and challenging, but the QALY approach at least provides a methodological framework to work from.

Building the QALY

The basic QALY

At its most simple, a QALY is a multiplication of the quantity of life experienced by the patient by a valuation of the quality of life they experienced. As we saw in *Chapter 6*, the valuation of a health state lends us a measure of **health utility**. So, the amount of time spent in a health state is then multiplied by the utility score given to that state.

- One year spent in perfect health (as perfect health has a utility score of 1) would give us 1 QALY.

- Equally, two years spent in a health state valued with a utility score of 0.5, would generate 1 QALY.

- A treatment which created 4 more years of survival, valued with a utility score of 0.25, would also generate 1 QALY.

In terms of outcomes, these options all generate 1 QALY and so would be considered equivalent.

> ### EXAMPLE 7.3 GENERATION OF QALYS
>
> Imagine two different treatments which improve survival by 8 years:
>
> Treatment A provides survival in a health state with a utility score of 0.25
>
> Treatment B provides survival in a health state with a utility score of 0.5
>
> In terms of QALYs gained, treatment A provides 2 QALYS (8 yrs x 0.25) whereas treatment B provides 4 QALYs (8 yrs x 0.5).
>
> So, treatment B generates 2 additional QALYs when compared to treatment A.

Example 7.3 shows the QALYs generated by two different treatment options. In this example, treatment B is preferable to treatment A, in terms of QALYs generated. It is important to note, though, that this comparison of treatments does not take into account any of the costs involved.

Real-life QALYs

As we all know, a person's health does change over time. A terminal cancer patient's survival wouldn't be in one health state: it would be in a number of different health states as their disease progressed.

Health economics is usually interested in the impact of a treatment on a patient over time, and for this analysis to truly reflect that patient's experience. So we really need to come up with a fair comparison of treatments, over the course of each specific treatment. We do this by comparing the health profile of a patient who is receiving the new treatment with a patient who is receiving the current standard care.

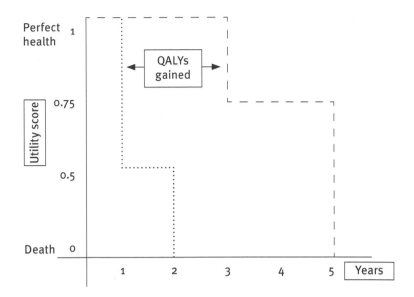

FIGURE 7.1 The dotted line represents the current standard of care, and the dashed line the new treatment. We can see that the new treatment doesn't just improve survival (death takes place later than with current treatment) but it also allows the patient to remain in a health state with a higher utility for longer. So you can see from the graph that the current standard of care generates 1 year at 1 QALY, and another year at half a QALY, so generates 1.5 QALYs. The new treatment offers 3 years at 1 QALY, then 2 years at 0.75 QALY, giving 4.5 QALYs.

This may not always be the case. There may be times when survival is extended, but at a reduced utility (a comatose patient on life support for example). In these cases, the QALY approach is very useful: if you were simply hoping to improve the survival of your patients, then you may recommend a treatment which doesn't improve the quality of life of your patients. In fact you could be recommending a treatment which some may consider to be detrimental.

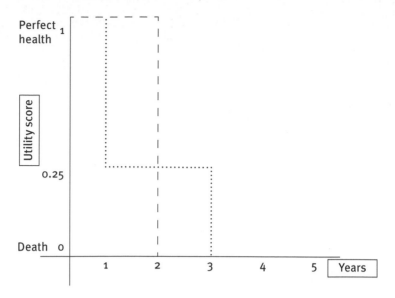

FIGURE 7.2 In this example, if we were only looking at survival, we may recommend the treatment which extended survival to three years. But this treatment only generates (1 × 1 QALY + 2 × 0.25 QALY) = 1.5 QALYs. The alternative treatment, whilst only offering 2 years of survival, does so at 1 QALY. So, 2 × 1 QALY = 2 QALYs, which may be preferable to the patient.

The QALY approach allows the decision-maker to have more information, which may lead them to look more broadly at the benefits of a treatment than just survival.

When QALYs aren't perfect

We can see how the use of a QALY can help to demonstrate the potential benefits of competing treatments as a combined measure of quality of life and overall survival. We must note, though, that they are not always a perfect measure of clinical outcomes, as *Example 7.4* demonstrates.

EXAMPLE 7.4 THE LIMITATIONS OF THE QALY

Say we have two different drugs; one is an injection, and the other is a tablet. Both have the same clinical benefits. Would a QALY detect a difference between these in terms of patient preferences (if any)?

Suppose the injection had to be given by trained medical staff, at a specialist centre, three times a week, but the tablet was simply taken twice a day with food.

The injection is likely to have a more severe impact on the patient's quality of life but there wouldn't be any difference between the two treatments in terms of a QALY analysis.

There are some cases where the use of a QALY will only generate a partial picture, because some very important health outcomes and effects can be overlooked:

- *Neurological conditions*
  In conditions such as Alzheimer's disease, where the patients themselves may not be well equipped to provide a utility measure.

- *Chronic disease*
  Here the quality of life someone experiences is of paramount importance and survival is of lower concern.

- *Preventative or health improvement schemes*
  The valuation placed on a health state is very much dependent upon that person's specific circumstances. For example, consider the case of a top class sports player, compared with an office worker, compared with a pensioner. The same health state (tennis elbow, for example) for each of them might elicit very different values.

There have been other criticisms of the QALY approach. Some economists and health physiologists believe that the QALY fails to place sufficient weight on emotional and mental health problems. It is also insensitive to the impact a health state can have on others who may care for the individual.

Equally, the question of whose health utility valuation of any particular health state is used as the basis for QALY analysis continues to provoke discussion. Should we use the general public's valuations, since healthcare is paid for by the tax payer in the UK, or should we take the valuation of the person who is experiencing the health state?

Often there are a large number of different factors which affect the outcome of a particular treatment and some argue that a QALY analysis cannot take all of these factors into account.

Also, by using population surveys, how sensitive are the generic instruments in capturing the true patient experience? Equally, do these patient surveys truly reflect the preferences of the population? It has often been suggested that the wider population would much prefer to treat a child than an elderly person if they were competing for the same resources. It has also been suggested that the wider population values improving severe health issues more than it does alleviating more mild conditions. Can a QALY demonstrate these preferences effectively?

There is a growing body of opinion that many of the QALYs used for comparison are too simplistic or generic, since QALYs are often developed from standard instruments (questionnaires). For example, the widely-used EQ-5D uses surveys of the general population to develop the utility weights. Critics say that this cannot be fully representative of the patient experience of their disease, as there is a growing weight of evidence to suggest that there is variation in disease between patients, which a generic instrument may fail to capture. With these comments in mind, many health economists are developing condition-specific instruments to help to build a QALY which is more sensitive to these variations.

What to watch out for...

QALYs can be very complex to understand at first, but I hope you can see now that they are simply a composite measure which is trying to account for the length of life, as well as the quality of life being experienced. So when reading papers which use the QALY, consider the following:

- How have the health utilities been assessed? It is always important to look at how the health utilities used have been assessed, and to examine the perspective of evaluation. Are these society's valuations, or the patient's? Neither is more correct (or incorrect) than the other, but it is important to be consistent in their application within a paper. If the utility weights are wrong, you can't rely on the QALYs calculated.

- Where has the assessment of length of life come from? Again, if this is not reliable, neither is the QALY value. Is the value from a peer-reviewed publication? Or from a robust well-conducted randomized controlled clinical trial? Clearly, these values would be more credible than using QALY values from a survey undertaken privately in a small group of people.

The use of QALYs in healthcare decision-making is becoming more and more widespread. Whilst it can be argued that there are flaws to this approach, it does allow a framework for commissioners to consistently compare treatments across competing patient groups when deciding on resource allocation. QALYs help commissioners to determine which new treatments have the greatest chance of delivering the maximum health benefits for their populations, given their limited healthcare budgets.

8 Cost utility analysis

The health economic Holy Grail?

What is it?

Cost utility analysis is a type of cost-effectiveness analysis. It is unique in that it uses life years saved, weighted for a valuation of the quality of life experienced during those years, as a health outcome measure. Those health outcome measures are called Quality-Adjusted Life Years (QALYs).

Introduction

Cost utility analysis is an analytical technique which health economists are using more and more– it's almost the default setting for a lot of health economists. At its core, cost utility analysis is very similar to the other techniques we have looked at; we are simply comparing the costs and benefits of one option with an alternative option. The difference here is that cost utility analysis relies heavily on the use of Quality-Adjusted Life Years (QALYs), as introduced in *Chapter 7*.

Cost utility analysis has an important place in health economic evaluation, as it allows a comparison of the value of different healthcare options, which may have very different healthcare benefits. By using the QALY we can make comparisons without having to place monetary values on a person's health-related quality of life, as we know this is fraught with problems and difficulty.

How important is this concept? ✪✪✪✪✪

Put simply, this evaluation method is really quite important, because it is becoming a 'gold standard' for health economic evaluations.

To refresh, a QALY is a measure of health which is a combination of the length of life experienced weighted against the health-related quality of life experienced. So, the QALY is the measure of benefit which is used in a cost utility analysis.

The outcome of a cost utility analysis is a **cost per QALY gained**, or in some cases the analysis can generate an **incremental cost-effectiveness ratio (ICER)**. This is the difference between the predicted costs of the two interventions, divided by the difference in the expected benefits; in this case, the difference in QALYs generated by the interventions.

Interestingly, often the results of a cost utility analysis are then compared to a **threshold ICER**. This is the limit which is set to allow or deny funding for, or approval of, the new healthcare technology under consideration. If the ICER is below the threshold set, then the proposal would generally be approved. If the ICER calculated is above the threshold ICER then more often than not, the new proposals are not approved. As a rule of thumb, the NHS in the UK uses a threshold of £30 000 per QALY, but this is a very loose generalization and does vary depending on circumstances (for example, if there is only one treatment available for a life-threatening condition then this threshold is often relaxed).

How easy is this idea to understand?

Cost utility analysis can be difficult to fully grasp if you are not confident in the use of the QALY. As the QALY is the main measure of benefit, this technique is reliant upon the tools used to generate the QALY measure. If we are not sure that the QALY is accurately capturing the patient experience, or if we are not confident that the QALY is truly representative of the value that society as a whole places on health improvements, then we may question the use and value of a cost utility analysis. As such, when reviewing a cost utility analysis, the construction of the QALY measures used is a key consideration.

As with any economic evaluation conducted in healthcare, a cost utility analysis in isolation is never quite enough to make a fully informed healthcare resource allocation decision, but it is a very useful technique and can really help to generate robust and informative analyses to assist in the decision-making process.

Should we always use a cost utility analysis?

As we have seen, there are many different approaches to economic evaluation in healthcare. All have their place, and while it may be tempting to think that the cost utility analysis is the approach which should be favoured, it isn't always appropriate or necessary. All the techniques we have discussed so far are valid and extremely useful; the different types of evaluation are defined by the way they approach the capturing of the measure of effect. Or more simply, how do they measure the benefit?

Now for some decisions it may very useful to measure the benefit a particular way. If we are comparing asthma treatments, then their effect on Forced Expiratory Volume (FEV1) may be a perfectly adequate outcome measure. Generating a QALY measure here may be unnecessary. As QALYs are a combination of the length of life experienced weighted by the health-related quality of life the patient experiences, it may be more appropriate to use cost utility analysis when the healthcare interventions under consideration are broad ranging, or may impact across a number of different healthcare activities.

A common criticism of the QALY approach is that it is too simplistic, as QALYs are often developed from standard instruments such as the EQ-5D, which uses surveys of the general population to develop the utility weights. Critics say that this cannot be fully representative of the patient experience of their disease; there is a growing weight of evidence to suggest that there is variation in disease between patients, which a generic instrument may fail to capture. With this comment in mind, many health economists are developing condition-specific instruments to help to build a QALY which is more sensitive to these variations.

Incremental Cost-Effectiveness Ratios (ICER)

Many cost utility analyses generate an incremental cost-effectiveness ratio (see *Example 4.2* for a reminder of this). This is calculated by taking the difference in costs between the health interventions under consideration and dividing this by the difference in QALYs generated by each intervention.

It is very compelling to think that we could conduct many cost utility analyses, comparing and analysing all sorts of different types of healthcare interventions and then build ourselves a 'league table' of all these results, placing the most cost-effective at the top and running right down to the least cost-effective at the bottom. Then budget holders would have the relatively simple job of just funding each of the interventions in turn, working their way down the table (starting by funding the intervention with the lowest cost per QALY), until finally they would simply run out of money, safe in the knowledge that they have maximized the health benefits given their restricted budget. Sounds lovely, doesn't it?

However, we have to be realistic. We will never be able to compare all the interventions with every other possible use of that money to improve health, nor would we want to. So what should we do with these cost utility analyses? The current approach is for decision-makers, be that the Department of Health or local decision-makers, to set a threshold. That is, the decision-makers establish their willingness to pay for health gain. This is commonly referred to as the threshold incremental cost-effectiveness ratio. As such, the decision to fund a new intervention is guided by whether or not the ICER generated by the cost utility analysis falls above or below this threshold ICER. If the analysis shows that the ICER generated falls above the threshold ICER, it is very unlikely to be funded. Sometimes this rule is relaxed as there may be no other alternative treatment available, but as a rule, if the ICER exceeds the threshold ICER then the technology isn't adopted.

Cost utility analyses are useful as they can overcome the issues of applying a standard cost benefit analysis to the world of healthcare. They allow the decision-makers to be able to compare the relative value of different healthcare interventions across disease areas, and across different health problems. As healthcare becomes more and more expensive, and as the populations of developed economies continue to age, these issues are becoming more and more relevant to examine. Because cost utility analyses are designed to compare different areas, they are extremely relevant when considering these challenges.

Thanks to bodies such as NICE, utilities and QALY weights are more and more prevalent and as such, the cost of conducting a cost utility analysis has come down in recent years as the requirement to collect prospective QALY data has diminished, and where it is required, the widespread availability of generic QALY instruments means this can be done affordably.

With this all said, it is important to note that with many healthcare interventions, there are a lot of different factors which have to be taken into consideration. The criticism levelled at the cost utility approach is simply, is it able to fully account for all these different factors which clearly have an effect on the outcomes? For example, say we have two different drugs; one is an injection, and the other is a tablet. Both have the same clinical benefits. Would a QALY detect a difference between these in terms of patient preferences (if these were to exist)? Also, by using population surveys, how sensitive are the generic instruments in capturing the true patient experience? Equally, do these patient surveys truly reflect the preferences of the population? It has often been suggested that the wider population would much prefer to treat a child than an elderly person if they were competing for the same resources. It has also been suggested that the wider population values improving severe health issues more than it does alleviating more mild conditions. Can a cost utility analysis find and test these assumptions adequately?

What to look out for...

As we have seen, the cost utility analysis is very closely linked to the use of the QALY. If we don't believe that the QALYs have been collected well, or calculated properly, then the whole analysis can be open to question. We must remember, though, that a cost utility analysis is very useful when choosing between different courses of action, especially when their benefits cannot be directly compared.

- Is the QALY a reliable unit on which to base health policy decisions? Is it repeatable? Utilities are currently measured by different techniques, and the results vary according to the method used.

- Differences in how preference weights are gathered can constrain the ability to credibly compare cost utility analyses where the effectiveness measure is presented in QALYs.

- Is the QALY measured in the study applicable to the population that will be influenced by the policy in question? We know that utility estimates vary according to who is making the estimate.

- Whose estimate of utility really is relevant to the decision to adopt the technology? There is still no unanimity as to whose viewpoint should be used when making policy decisions.

So, a well-performed cost utility analysis is always a great start, and is always a highly important piece of information to use to inform a healthcare allocation decision. It just isn't the **only** piece of information required. We've seen that this type of analysis can often fail to capture a number of factors which could be very influential on the final allocation decision and what it does take into consideration, it does so with varying degrees of sensitivity.

However, when reviewing cost utility analyses, we must check the assumptions regarding the QALY weights first, and then look to see if all the other assumptions in the analysis seem fair. A cost utility analysis, when conducted well, is extremely helpful to healthcare decision-makers.

9 Evidence-based medicine

But isn't all medicine evidence-based...?

What is it?

Evidence-based medicine (EBM) is the practice of medicine (or the use of healthcare interventions) as guided by, or based upon, clinical expertise clearly supported by well-conducted scientific evidence. In addition, evidence-based medicine actively seeks to avoid the use of those interventions shown by scientific evidence to be less efficacious or even harmful.

Introduction

The objective of EBM is to ensure the integration of the appropriate clinical expertise and patient values, along with the best research evidence, right into the heart of the decision-making process for healthcare.

Good doctors always use both their individual clinical expertise alongside the best available external evidence. We should note that for EBM, neither of these resources on its own is enough. Without the application of clinical expertise, there is the risk that even excellent external evidence advocating use of a specific treatment may not be appropriate for an individual patient. However, without the use of the current best available evidence, healthcare practice runs the risk of becoming outdated, to the detriment of patients.

How important is this concept? ✪✪✪✪✪

The basic concept of evidence-based medicine is that **we should treat where there is evidence of benefit, and not treat where there is evidence of no benefit, or even harm**. When it's put down like that it seems very intuitive, doesn't it?

However, any economic analysis is only as good as the data which have gone into it. It's the old 'garbage in, garbage out' rule.

So what is a good evidence base for medical technologies? Medical interventions were starting to be formally assessed by clinical trials in the early 1940s as there was a recognition that, just because something was thought to be beneficial, it didn't necessarily mean that it actually *was* beneficial. But the practice of reviewing the evidence and assessing the benefits of medical treatments is still a relatively new concept.

It wasn't until 1992 that the UK government invested in setting up the Cochrane Centre in Oxford with the clear objective of reviewing the wealth of available clinical data, by means of systematic reviews (which we will discuss in more detail in *Chapter 11*). There are now approximately 13 international centres within the Cochrane collaboration, and they are clearly an important force in developing evidence-based medicine throughout the world.

How easy is this idea to understand?

EBM is a pretty simple idea, and a reassuring one, too. Of course, nobody would want to use a drug or health technology which has not been fully tested, or one which doesn't have any evidence to show that it works well and provides benefit. Evidence-based medicine is a formalized approach to establish whether or not the evidence supports the use of a medicine or health intervention for a particular patient group, disease or condition.

There are a number of different sources we can use to establish the evidence:

- Personal clinical experience, 'Did the drug work well in treating this disease last time?'

- From colleagues, asking if they have used the drug before and, if so, how it performed.

- But more formally, we should be looking to the **published clinical literature** to provide the bedrock of the data.

It's important to recognize that the published clinical literature is a more robust level of evidence than personal experience. Clinical trials are often based upon many people's experiences as opposed to just personal experience.

In health economics (and remember that economics is all about the allocation of scarce resources), if we know which evidence base is more reliable, then we can use this evidence to reduce the amount of ineffective and often unnecessary prescribing done in healthcare today.

When should this be used?

Ideally, all healthcare professionals should be employing the principles of EBM every day. That said, it's not always easy to find the appropriate evidence in many cases. However, the internet has made the process of finding the relevant clinical literature much easier.

The Cochrane library is a great starting point (www. thecochranelibrary.com). This resource contains a lot of very high quality clinical evidence which is primarily designed to inform those people who have to make clinical decisions every day. It has multiple databases, all of which can be searched easily and quickly. It is a free access site for anyone who lives in the UK and I recommend this as a starting point, to dip your toe into the world of evidence-based medicine.

There are other sources of information too. Medline (www.pubmed. gov) hosts a wealth of clinical data but there is no quality grading applied here. It is simply a reporting of clinical papers, so some care needs to be taken.

Clinical evidence can be, and is, published and presented in a number of different forms. It's important to fully understand these different types, and where they rank on the **hierarchy of evidence**. Although there really isn't a single hierarchy of evidence which is accepted by all, what we do find is that there is a broad agreement on the relative strengths and weaknesses of the principal types of clinical research undertaken.

As a rule of thumb, *Box 9.1* shows a widely accepted hierarchy of evidence. This is not definitive, nor is it exhaustive, but it gives an idea as to how we can rank our evidence sources, going from strongest to weakest:

BOX 9.1 HIERARCHY OF EVIDENCE

1. Systematic reviews and meta-analyses
2. Well-conducted randomized controlled trials (RCTs)
3. Cohort studies
4. Case-control studies
5. Cross-sectional surveys
6. Case reports
7. Expert opinion/anecdotal experience

Generally, systematic review evidence and meta-analyses (more on these in *Chapter 11*) are considered the best form of evidence (it can be argued that as these techniques often combine data from multiple well-conducted randomized controlled trials (RCTs), and can also include data from other study types as well, they represent a more rigorous level of evidence than a single RCT). Randomized controlled trials are usually considered the next rung down the ladder and normally rank above observational studies. Expert opinions and any anecdotal experiences are almost always ranked at the bottom.

Understanding the approach undertaken by exponents of evidence-based medicine is important when thinking about health economic analysis. You should consider the strength of the evidence which has been used to inform the model parameters and assess whether or not the model is appropriate, robust and informative to your decision. The adoption of evidence-based medicine is still increasing, and it is becoming a well-recognized tool in the process of commissioning new healthcare services globally. The techniques of evidence-based medicine are being applied to all aspects of healthcare delivery, not just to drugs and medical devices, but also to surgical techniques, diagnostics and to lifestyle choices.

Thanks to the internet and modern communication systems, clinicians are more and more able to use evidence-based medicine principles in their everyday practice. This helps to make sure that the right treatment is given to the right patient, for the right reasons, more often. If we can achieve this, then clearly this practice will have economic benefits as well. It is obviously very inefficient to prescribe an inappropriate treatment initially, and to then have to prescribe a second, more appropriate treatment down the line. Practising evidence-based medicine can help to avoid these types of inefficiencies.

What to look out for...

- How strong is the study design?
- How many patients were recruited into the study?

- Does this study represent my patient?

- Who sponsored/paid for the research?

As there is no universal agreement on the hierarchy of evidence, always review any paper to see which evidence type they are placing at the top. Do you agree? Sometimes an RCT can be less relevant than a well-conducted systematic review (which we will cover in *Chapter 11*). Equally, understanding who funded the study may help identify any potential biases which may be present in the analysis.

Even though the concept of evidence-based medicine is compelling, not all are aware of it, or consistently practise it. One potential pitfall is that some patients and members of the public may take its application for granted, assuming that this process is the basis for all decisions in healthcare; this isn't always the case, as we have seen.

We should recognize that patients are probably not aware of how evidence-based medicine principles can impact on their specific treatment – for example, when a new study shows that a drug treatment is no longer considered effective for their particular circumstances. Occasionally the evidence will show that a therapy is not providing benefits and as such, should no longer be prescribed. This has nothing to do with its price (although if a therapy is ineffective, then it is highly unlikely to be cost-effective!) but simply a rationalization of healthcare provision, ensuring that the most appropriate therapies are prescribed.

10 Critical appraisal

I don't believe it!

What is it?

Critical appraisal involves the use of clearly defined, transparent methodologies to appraise the data presented in published research. Critical appraisal methods are a key component of the systematic review process (covered in more detail in *Chapter 11*). These methods are also widely used when applying evidence-based healthcare to inform clinical decision-making.

Introduction

Clinical research is the basis of most health economics models. Critical appraisal means interpreting the strengths and weaknesses of the research. It is not a negative dismissal of a piece of clinical research, nor is it simply an assessment of the results alone. Critical appraisal is a balanced assessment which considers:

- the strengths of a piece of research

- the research process used

- the results achieved.

> ## EXAMPLE 10.1 THE CRITICAL APPRAISAL PROCESS
>
> Imagine that in the early noughties, a rental company decided to build some new office blocks, to rent out. All of the offices were identical workspaces, with high specification interiors, and identical facilities, in a much sought-after business location. Once finished, there was initially a lot of interest in the offices but after three months not one of them had been let. When the company asked the potential renters why they had chosen to not rent one of the offices, they were always told that there was nothing wrong with the offices, but that the offices didn't have a 'good feel' about them.
>
> A member of the rental company's staff had recently completed a course in feng shui and suggested to the directors that they refit the offices, closely following the feng shui principles. Deciding there was nothing to lose, as none of the units had been let, the company refurbished three of the offices using these principles, whilst the remaining three remained in their original state.
>
> All three of the refitted offices were let as soon as the refit was complete. The rental company decided that after this controlled experiment they would ensure that all future office developments of theirs would be designed using feng shui principles.
>
> (With thanks to Shropshire health libraries for the inspiration for this example)

Unsurprisingly, *Example 10.1* is not a reliable piece of research; here are a few thoughts as to why.

- The sample size is very small

- Were the refitted offices refitted with newer/better desks and furniture? Could this have been more attractive to the potential tenants?

- Were the refitted offices chosen at random? Maybe the refitted offices were on the top floor, which may have been more appealing?

- Were the prospective tenants told that the offices had been redesigned according to feng shui principles? (i.e. were they blinded?) For some this could have been enticement enough to rent...

From this example, therefore, it is not possible to conclude that feng shui was effective in selling the offices. Hopefully you can see from this the real value of critical appraisal to health care economics – it is vital that the data we are using in our models are as reliable and accurate as possible; critical appraisal helps us to assess the reliability of these data.

How important is this concept? ✪ ✪ ✪ ✪ ✪

Critical appraisal is another technique which is an integral part of the practice of evidence-based medicine. Critical appraisal is a process which carefully examines clinical data and research in a systematic fashion, and then judges these data on their overall reliability, value and trustworthiness in a specific clinical context. You should always be assessing the 'worth' or 'value' of any piece of information or evidence you look at.

Clearly these skills are not something that we can cover completely within one chapter. It can take a long time for a reviewer to become fully adept in the skills of critical appraisal, and to be able to make full sense of the scientific literature. What we can do here though is introduce the key concepts, so that you are able to value and judge clinical papers to a degree yourselves.

The main concept I hope to explore here is that all studies are subject to **bias**. Different study designs are employed simply to try to minimize these inherent biases. The correct study design for the research topic in question is one in which the bias is minimized.

How easy is this idea to understand?

There is quite a lot to get to grips with here. People dedicate their professional careers to becoming fully skilled in critical appraisal. The detailed analysis can be very complex indeed, but the principle of critical appraisal is more straightforward.

When is this type of analysis used?

Personally, I think that everyone would want to enjoy the best possible health that they can. It is becoming apparent that to be able to achieve this we need good reliable scientific information about what might help (or what might hinder) our bid for better health.

To try to answer these questions, research is conducted and the results are then collated and analysed to produce some hopefully useful and meaningful information. A key point you need to remember is that not all of the results generated are of good quality. It is also true that sometimes studies are published with misleading results or even results which are untrue. A classic example of this is the study linking MMR with autism which was originally published in the *Lancet*, but has since been clearly proven to be wrong and was declared fraudulent by the *BMJ* in 2011. Understandably, we need to be able to differentiate the great studies from those which are simply misleading, unhelpful, or untruthful.

So critical appraisal techniques are tools which enable us to tell whether or not a piece of clinical research has been performed well, and whether or not the results reported are valid and useful.

We need to be able to look at a piece of clinical evidence and be able to decide if the information has been generated in a way which makes the findings reliable. We also need to be able to understand and apply the results correctly and be confident that the results are applicable to the clinical context we are considering.

Critical appraisal – the basics

Bias

When we are critically appraising clinical research, it is very important for us to first look for any sources of **bias** which may be affecting the study. Is there anything which may have affected the results of the study?

Generally all studies are subject to some form of bias. Different study designs are employed simply to try to minimize these inherent biases. The correct study design for the research topic in question is always the one in which the bias is minimized. Let's look at the three broad types of bias which may be present in a study.

Selection bias

The selection of patients into a study, or their allocation to a particular treatment group may produce a sample that is not truly representative of the general population, or it may create treatment groups that are systematically different. This would mean that any treatment effects highlighted by the study may not be replicated in the general population, as the study does not reflect the general population. A randomized controlled trial is the key to avoiding this bias.

Measurement bias

Sometimes the measurement of outcomes in a study is not performed well. This may be caused by an inaccuracy in the measurement instrument, or by a bias in the expectations of patients in the study or even carers or researchers, which we will explore more later in this chapter. This effect may be addressed by making sure participants, carers or researchers do not know whether or not they are taking the new drug; this process is called **blinding**.

Analysis bias

The protection against bias that randomization infers can only be maintained if all the study participants remain in the group to which they were originally allocated and also complete their follow-up. Any participants who change groups, or withdraw from the study or are perhaps lost to follow-up may be systematically different from those who complete the study. This again means that the results will not be fully generalizable to the general population. This analysis bias can be reduced by maximizing follow-up and evaluating *all* the patients who entered the study (you may see this referred to as an **Intention to Treat analysis**).

Hierarchy of evidence

As we discussed in *Chapter 9*, there is a generally accepted hierarchy of evidence. This list is not definitive, nor is it exhaustive, but it gives an idea as to how you could rank your evidence sources, going from strongest to weakest.

BOX 10.1 HIERARCHY OF EVIDENCE

1. Systematic reviews and meta-analysis
2. Well-conducted randomized controlled trials (RCTs)
3. Cohort studies
4. Case-control studies
5. Cross-sectional surveys
6. Case reports
7. Expert opinion/anecdotal experience

Systematic reviews and meta-analysis

At the top, systematic reviews and meta-analysis are considered to be the highest level of evidence, if conducted properly. These will be discussed in more depth in *Chapter 11*, so I won't spoil the surprise here.

Randomized controlled trial

A randomized controlled trial (RCT) is made up of a 'treatment' group and a 'control' group. The treatment group will be exposed to the treatment under investigation, whilst the control group will not. The key element here is that membership of each group is decided randomly. There is no bias as to who will receive the new technology or the standard treatment. This means that the only effect we should see should be a direct result of the change in treatment.

Sometimes, to further reduce bias, blinding will be used as well, as we briefly discussed earlier. This is so that the patients themselves do not know whether or not they are receiving the new treatment. In addition, there may be a second level of blinding (often called double-blinding) so that the researchers do not know which group has received the new treatment either.

Why do we do this? Well, it is thought that patients may report a different experience if they know they are trying a new or experimental drug. This is often the case if the disease being treated is terminal. Equally, researchers who know which group is receiving the new treatment may look harder for differences to support the use of the new drug than they would if they didn't know which group was which. This means that, with blinding, if there is a difference found we are far more confident that there truly is a difference.

That said, not all interventions lend themselves well to an RCT design. Drugs when compared to a placebo do; surgical interventions or implantations do not. It's very hard to blind a patient to having had an operation, or to blind a surgeon to performing one!

Also, RCTs can be very, very expensive to run and in order to show fairly small degrees of difference between interventions, we often need to recruit thousands and thousands of patients.

Cohort studies

Cohort studies follow two groups of people over time. Normally the comparison is between one of the groups receiving a specific treatment, whilst the other group does not. Sometimes the comparison is made between a group which has been exposed to something, whilst the other group has not – studies of the effects of smoking are classic examples of this.

It is important that the two groups we are comparing are as closely matched as possible, apart from the treatment or exposure, so we can be sure that any differences seen can be attributed to that, and not to some other confounding factor. The groups are followed over time, so that hopefully we get consistent and sustained results. If run correctly, cohort studies can be very useful in identifying healthcare impacts.

Case control studies

Case control studies also have a place. These types of studies are mainly used for causation studies, where a patient with a particular health outcome is matched to a patient without this as a control. Investigations are then made into possible causes in both of the patients. For example, further data may then be collected on those individuals and the two groups are compared to find out if other characteristics found (again perhaps a history of smoking) are also different between the two groups. Whilst not the most robust of designs, this can often be the only option in very rare conditions. For example, we may have a group of patients with a very rare form of cancer; we could match these patients with another group matched in as many ways as possible apart from the rare cancer. We could then examine their histories to try to establish if there were any common causal factors shared by the rare cancer group which weren't present in the matched control group.

There are also lesser forms of evidence published; for some interventions/exposures/conditions these can often be the only form of study available. You might see terms such as: case studies; case series or even cross-sectional surveys – you don't particularly need to know the ins and outs of these but you should bear in mind that the evidence from these studies is not as reliable as that from the studies detailed above.

What to look out for...

There are checklists available which you can use to help you to critically appraise the evidence you are reviewing. There are different checklists for the different types of studies you are looking at: RCTs, systematic reviews and so on. These checklists are great as they can really help you to focus on the most important aspects of the article.

Two great sources for these checklists are:
Scottish Intercollegiate Guideline Network
http://www.sign.ac.uk/methodology/checklists.html
and

The Centre for Evidence Based Medicine
http://www.cebm.net/index.aspx?o=1157

They are excellent resources and I strongly suggest you make use of them.

The checklists enable us to answer the key questions:

- What are the results?

- Are they significant?

- Are the results valid?

- How was the research conducted?

- How will these results help my work with patients?

Further questions we should always ask of any research include:

- Does this information tell me anything new?

- Is this applicable to my patients?

- Should I act on this information if it suggests I should change my current practice?

11 Systematic reviews and meta-analyses

'A wise man... proportions his belief to the evidence.'

David Hume 1711–1776

What are they?

Systematic reviews and **meta-analyses** are techniques which bring together multiple studies and sources of evidence to try to deliver stronger, more robust conclusions on the effectiveness of a treatment. This is why both are covered together in this chapter.

A systematic review is simply a review of the literature which relates to a specific and focused research question. The aim is to identify, appraise, evaluate, select and finally synthesize all the good quality research evidence which is available and relevant to that question.

A meta-analysis is a statistical method which is used to combine the results of a number of different, independent studies to generate a larger sample size for evaluation and therefore allows us to draw a stronger conclusion than can be provided by any single study in isolation.

Introduction

There has been a clear increase in the number of medical, health economic and healthcare papers published over the last 50 years. This increase in evidence generation shows no signs of slowing down. This fact makes keeping on top of the primary research evidence available to you an impossible task. There simply are not enough hours in the day to do so. At the same time, there has been a revolution in terms of access to medical articles via the internet. A search for a particular subject can create a somewhat intimidating number of hits to review. In addition to the wealth of information, there is the new issue of developing and maintaining the skills required to fully master the wide array of electronic media which enables this access to unfeasibly large amounts of medical information.

Increasingly, everyone involved with healthcare, from clinicians and nurses through to patients and their families, now have much higher medical information needs than they did 30 years ago; that is, these groups are looking for good quality evidence on the effectiveness and appropriateness of a wide range of different healthcare technologies, not just a few. For a lot of clinicians, this requirement is in direct conflict with their hectic professional lives, and cannot come at the expense of patient time. For patients, the volume of information can be overpowering. Couple this with a lack of expert knowledge and this can often lead to patients requesting treatments based wholly upon unreliable information, which creates many unnecessary conflicts, and could be detrimental to patient care.

In health economics terms, we need to know which evidence we should be using when deciding on the appropriate treatment options – systematic reviews and meta-analysis are both tools which help find the best evidence.

How important are these concepts? ✪✪✪✪✪

In general, systematic reviews are useful to clearly establish the clinical and cost-effectiveness of a particular treatment. A single study does not always convince in isolation. More and more, systematic reviews are an essential step to clearly showing if a technology or treatment is feasible, or if it is appropriate in a particular case (ethically or culturally), or if it offers additional benefits over an existing treatment option. Systematic reviews of high quality randomized controlled trials are crucial to evidence-based medicine. Systematic reviews of all evidence sources are also highly valuable. An understanding of systematic reviews and how to implement them in practice is becoming mandatory for all professionals involved in the delivery of healthcare.

Meta-analysis provides a specific estimate of treatment effect to be expected, giving due weight to the size of the different studies included in the analysis. It is another form of systematic analysis which makes use of multiple studies or evaluations in order to draw general conclusions, develop support for hypotheses, and/or produce an estimate of overall programme effects.

How easy are these ideas to understand?
👍👍👍👍👍

Conceptually, these are simple ideas. We look at the published data, and then we identify all the papers which relate to our research question and pull them out for review. However, undertaking such a task is really no small commitment. It is an awful lot of hard work, especially when trying to identify all of the relevant papers, and it is vital to understand whether or not they are relevant to your question.

Systematic review methodology really is the cornerstone of any meta-analysis. It is absolutely vital to be certain that you have identified all the relevant studies (both published and unpublished, if the latter are available from authors and/or researchers) which are available to you, and to then evaluate the quality of each study, both in terms of the design employed and the execution of each study. The objective of systematic reviews is to present a balanced and impartial summary of the existing research, enabling decisions on effectiveness to be based on all the relevant studies of a sufficient quality.

When is this type of analysis used?

Systematic reviews are clearly required when there is an important clinical question to answer. Perhaps there have been several primary studies published – it may well be that these studies all have incongruent findings – and this would also mean that there is substantial uncertainty regarding the most beneficial and appropriate treatment.

Meta-analysis presents the reviewer with a logical and useful way of dealing with multiple studies which could be confusing for anyone who is trying to make practice decisions using evidence-based research.

Systematic reviews

Systematic reviews of high-quality randomized controlled trials are crucial to evidence-based medicine. Systematic reviews of all evidence sources are also highly valuable. An understanding of systematic reviews and how to implement them in practice is becoming mandatory for all professionals involved in the delivery of health care. Systematic reviews are not limited to medicine and are quite common in other sciences.

Systematic reviews are used to:

- inform future research, especially if the options for treatment may be unclear or current approaches have been unable to answer a clinical issue

- secure research grant resources for clinical authors for primary healthcare studies

- evaluate healthcare technologies within the NHS in England and Wales. Systematic reviews are integral to both the multiple technology appraisals which NICE conducts and their single technology appraisal process.

It's clear that we have to apply very strict rules and criteria when we are conducting a systematic review. Fortunately, there is a formal process to help us. A basic understanding of the approach and steps taken to minimize bias can really help us when deciding if any given systematic review is well conducted. This will help us to evaluate whether or not we should change our practice and act upon their findings. One thing to look for is that in an ideal world, process of review should be undertaken according to a peer-reviewed protocol.

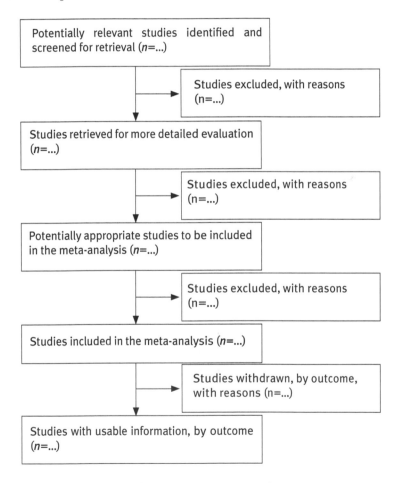

FIGURE 11.1 A current best practice protocol for systematic review. The individual steps are discussed below.

The first step is to frame an appropriate healthcare question. What exactly is it you are looking to establish or find out? You must start out with a clear idea of the objectives of your review. Which intervention are you looking at? Which patient group? Is there a specific sub-population you are interested in? Which types of evidence will you include? All studies ideally should be included if you believe that they will help answer the question. Equally, you should always be looking to ensure that the outcomes reported are appropriate to your question.

When you start to look in the literature, you need to search carefully for all the appropriate papers which relate to the activity in question. To avoid bias, this search of the literature must try to cover ALL the evidence databases, not just MEDLINE! To be thorough, certain journals are often hand-searched when necessary. Searching for the papers is no small task.

Once we have all the possible studies identified and available, then we can start the task of assessing them. Each study needs to be assessed for eligibility against the inclusion criteria set by the initial protocol, and full text papers can then be ordered for those papers which meet the criteria.

The studies which made the grade are then assessed for methodological quality, using a critical appraisal framework (as discussed in *Chapter 10*). As you can expect, any poor quality studies are discounted here but are usually discussed in the review report to demonstrate that they were identified and excluded.

With the final batch of studies in our hand, we then read them all and report their findings via a data extraction form. Even at this point in the process, some studies can be excluded. A final list of included studies is then created. To be really very rigorous, to try to further avoid bias, the assessment should ideally be conducted by two independent reviewers.

So, now we have completed data extraction forms, the findings from all the individual studies must be aggregated to produce an 'outcome'; an answer on whether or not the intervention you have looked at is useful or not in the context you predefined.

Meta-analysis

A meta-analysis, at its most simple, combines the results of several studies to generate a more robust measure of treatment effect. The technique involves a series of quite complex statistical calculations across the quantitative evidence that has been gathered (often from a systematic review). The exact details of these calculations are well beyond the scope of this book; when presented with evidence you simply need to be reassured that a meta-analysis has been performed.

Generally the role of a meta-analysis is to combine and to compare the statistical data reported by studies and to investigate if there are any large (unexpected) differences between all the research which has been identified. The meta-analysis approach allows us to make the best use of all the information we have gathered in our systematic review. By statistically combining the results of similar studies we can improve the precision of our estimates of treatment effect, and assess whether treatment effects are the same in similar situations. We have to take care to decide whether or not the results of individual studies are similar enough to be combined in a meta-analysis, because if they are not, this can affect the validity of the result.

There are many approaches to meta-analysis. It is important to note that meta-analysis is not simply a matter of adding up numbers of participants across studies. Remember that meta-analysis provide a specific estimate of the treatment effect which can be expected, giving due weight to the size of the different studies included in the analysis, not just an aggregation of all the studies.

What to look out for...

We have to be clear here that not every published systematic review is well conducted, rigorous and unbiased. The reader will want to scrutinize any review that purports to be systematic, to look for any possible limitations and to help them to decide if the outcomes and recommendations found should be applied to their clinical practice.

There are some questions we can ask of any paper to check its integrity as a good systematic review:

- Is the topic under question well defined?

- Was the search for papers conducted thoroughly?

- Was each study assessed for quality by independent or blinded reviewers?

- Were the criteria for the inclusion of the studies clearly described and applied?

- Was any missing information identified sought from the original study authors?

- Are the recommendations presented based firmly on the quality of the evidence?

- Was the role of chance investigated?

- Were the overall findings of the review assessed? Are they robust?

- Do the studies included in the review appear to indicate similar effects? If not, in the case of clinical effectiveness, was the heterogeneity of effect investigated, assessed and discussed?

There is always a danger of bias if we don't include all the relevant studies available in the review. A simple review, which may only include a number of the relevant papers, may be more likely to only report the positive outcomes.

Often, it is easier to publish positive papers in the higher impact journals than to publish papers which show no significant differences; so if you limited your search, you may only find positive papers. Informal reviews may also be tainted by the prior beliefs of the author. One of the strengths of a meta-analysis performed well on a rigorous systematic review is that it can easily overcome such issues and present an unbiased summary of the data available.

12 Health technology assessment in the UK

Identifying value, or rationing by another name?

What is it?

Health technology assessment (HTA), or appraisal, is a field of research which broadly focuses on evaluating and, on occasion, informing decisions made around governmental or healthcare policy.

Introduction

Initially, HTA methods were developed to provide a framework to bring together the two worlds of clinical research and policy-making in healthcare. Today, HTAs are conducted in many different countries around the world, and this practice continues to grow, driven by the desire to support the sometimes difficult and confusing policy decisions required in modern healthcare.

Broadly speaking, HTA reviews and assesses the current clinical, economic, social and ethical implications of the adoption (or cessation) of a treatment, in comparison to an agreed alternative course of action.

What sort of questions can HTA be used to address?

HTA is all about trying to define the relative value of a health technology, while taking into account the broadest possible scope of costs and benefits the technology might accrue. So, in theory, HTA methodologies should be able to address any health policy decision being faced.

However, HTA is not an exact science as a number of value judgements have to be applied to the process. HTA generally focuses on 'the value' (both the clinical and economic benefits) of the adoption of the technology in question, in comparison with current (or best) clinical practice.

Historically, HTA has generally addressed two issues:

- Clinical effectiveness – how well does this treatment work? Or more formally, how do the health outcomes generated by the appropriate application of the technology compare with the outcomes generated by the currently available technology alternatives?

- Cost-effectiveness – is it worth the money? Or again more formally, can we say that the improvements in health outcomes provided are proportionate to the extra costs associated with the adoption of the new technology? As we know from earlier, this is often decided using the QALY measure.

In these circumstances, HTA is used to help policy-makers decide which technologies truly are effective in both clinical and cost terms and which simply are not. But what makes the grade will vary from case to case, and country to country (see *Chapter 8*).

HTA also plays another role, by being able to help define the most appropriate circumstance, or patient group, for a particular treatment. At its best, HTA can lessen, or even stop, the use of health technologies which are proven to be dangerous and ineffective. Equally, by using HTA, we can identify those technologies whose cost is simply too high when compared with the benefits they bring.

It would be fair to say that most international HTA activity to date has focused on the assessment of new and in the most part, expensive pharmaceuticals being launched onto the market.

How important is this concept?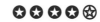

HTA is here to stay, in one form or another. Healthcare costs continue to rise whilst healthcare budgets are squeezed. In general people are living longer and the new technologies which are being developed tend to be either high cost products or niche products for a very specific condition. So, the need to evaluate the true 'value' of these new technologies has never been greater.

How easy is this idea to understand?

HTA is where all the concepts, techniques and ideas we have been exploring in this book come together. So, understandably this area can be rather tricky.

The different HTA bodies around the world all apply slightly different methodologies, and with good reason, as each country's healthcare system is structured in a slightly different way, and of course, the population demographics may be different. Different types of health technologies clearly require different types of clinical trials and different study designs, as we have already encountered, so the evidence base often dictates the HTA approach.

HTA in the UK

The use of HTA in the UK is not as new as you may think. In 1993, the National Coordinating Centre was set up by a group based at the University of Southampton (now called the National Institute for Health Research – www.hta.ac.uk). Ever since the inception of this centre, the UK has enjoyed a highly dynamic academic HTA programme which is well respected internationally. However, recently the term HTA has become heavily associated with the work of the National Institute for Health and Clinical Excellence (NICE) in England and Wales, although we should also note here that both Scotland and Wales have their own HTA agencies, the Scottish Medicines Consortium (SMC) and the All Wales Medicines Strategy Group (AWMSG), respectively.

The National Institute for Health and Clinical Excellence (www.nice.org.uk)

NICE started life back in 1999 when it was set up as an NHS special health authority. NICE has the responsibility of providing clear and implementable national guidance on the promotion of good health and the prevention and treatment of poor health.

The initial objective of the HTA work conducted by NICE was to produce clear national guidance on the value of specific health technologies, which included both pharmaceuticals and medical devices. NICE also wanted to appraise best clinical practice, through its clinical guidelines development processes. NICE is structured over three different centres working on their own remits: the Centre for Health Technology Evaluation; the Centre for Public Health Excellence; and the Centre for Clinical Practice. The Centre for Public Health Excellence was established in April 2005 and is pivotal in developing the NICE guidance on the promotion of good health and disease prevention.

We should note that when NICE was first publishing its guidance, it was purely in an advisory manner. However, this changed in January 2002; since then it has been mandatory for the NHS in England and Wales to provide funding for the interventions and treatment options recommended by NICE through its technology appraisal programme. In addition to this, all NHS organizations must review and take into consideration all their clinical management protocols following the publication of NICE's clinical guidelines.

Scottish Medicines Consortium (www.scottishmedicines.org.uk)

The Scottish Medicines Consortium began its work in January 2002. It is now part of NHS Quality Improvement Scotland and the remit of the SMC is to assess the incremental value of all the newly licensed pharmaceuticals, all of the new formulations of current medicines and any substantial new use for established medicines in terms of their 'value for money' when used in the NHS in Scotland.

The SMC differs from NICE in that it currently doesn't assess medical devices and it assesses new pharmaceuticals or new indications for medicines at the time of launch, whereas NICE often assesses products at any time. The SMC hopes to issue its guidance to NHS Scotland within 12 weeks of the products being made available to patients. If a product demonstrates that it is good value for money, and is approved by the SMC, it is automatically included onto the area drugs and therapeutics committee (ADTC) formularies in Scotland. Being included here means that the medicine approved is allowed to be prescribed on the NHS in Scotland. Conversely, if a medicine is not recommended by the SMC, it simply will not be included on the ADTC formularies and, as a result, access to the product will be strictly limited.

It is important for us to note that the healthcare provision in Scotland is devolved, and the regional health boards are responsible for providing care. Although NHS Scotland is funded centrally from the UK Department of Health, NHS Scotland is responsible for managing the allocation of healthcare funding to the nine health boards within Scotland. These health boards are responsible for providing healthcare to their area's population. Each of these health boards has its own ADTC, as mentioned above.

All Wales Medicines Strategy Group (www.wales.nhs.uk/awmsg)

At around the same time as the SMC was established, the All Wales Medicines Strategy Group was set up to advise the Welsh Assembly of any advances in healthcare, in order to help the Assembly with its strategic planning. The remit of the AWMSG is to develop timely, independent and authoritative guidance on the use of new pharmaceuticals, and to inform the Assembly about the cost implications of adopting these medicines for routine use on the NHS in Wales. In addition, the AWMSG advises the Assembly on its prescribing strategy for Wales.

The AWMSG aims to make its recommendations soon after the launch of a product, much like the SMC, and it hopes to produce its guidance within 18 months of a company notifying them of any new developments. However, as NICE guidance also covers Wales, the AWMSG will not consider appraising a pharmaceutical if NICE intends to publish its appraisal of the same product within 18 months.

To begin with, the AWMSG process focused purely on assessing high-cost medicines (the AWMSG defined these as medicines which cost more than £2000 per patient per year), but recently they have started to broaden their scope to other medicines below this threshold and they do have plans to review all the new indications.

How do some technologies end up being appraised by NICE, and others do not?

NICE does not operate in quite the same way as SMC and AWMSG. The main difference is that NICE does not evaluate every new treatment when it comes on to the market. NICE argues that this workload would simply be too much for it. It selects which treatments it will review according to the specific criteria set out below.

- Is the treatment, if adopted, likely to result in a significant health benefit, taken across the NHS as a whole, if given to all patients for whom it is indicated?

- Is the treatment likely to create a significant impact on other health-related government policies (for example, reduction in health inequalities)?

- Is the treatment likely to make a significant impact on NHS resources (financial or otherwise) if made available to all patients for whom it is indicated?

- Is a NICE review likely to be able to add value? For instance, if NICE were to not produce guidance, could there be significant controversy or confusion regarding the interpretation or significance of the available evidence on clinical and cost-effectiveness?

NICE publishing guidance is important, but actually changing practice is a different matter.

It has been over a decade since the first NICE guidance was published, and as often reported in the media, the implementation of NICE guidance remains patchy and uneven across the NHS as a whole. This has continued to be an issue despite the fact that any guidance published by NICE following a technology appraisal by the Institute is mandatory on the NHS, and there are clear Department of Health policies stating that the findings should be implemented within three months.

This is a disappointing outcome as NICE was initially created to ultimately reduce variations in the adoption of new technologies by area (to try to solve the spectre of 'post code rationing'). NICE is aware of these issues and has established an internal working group to try to help with the implementation of its guidance, but as we still see in the UK, full implementation remains very difficult to achieve.

Glossary

Allocative efficiency

A methodology in which resources are distributed for the widest possible benefit; any change in the allocation of these resources would then result in a reduction in net benefits. One example is a programme where the allocation of resources is such that no change in spending priorities could improve the welfare of one person without reducing the welfare of another.

Average cost-effectiveness – *see* **Cost**

Benefits

The total sum of the effects on wellbeing (can be positive or negative) which a particular programme generates. Some of these benefits, such as relief of pain or suffering, can be difficult to quantify.

Bias

Any trend in the collection, analysis, interpretation, publication or review of data that can lead to conclusions that are systematically different from the truth. In a clinical trial, bias refers to the effects on a conclusion that may be incorrect. For example, when a researcher or patient knows what treatment is being given, this may affect their view of the outcome of the treatment.

Blinding

The concealment of information about which group a patient enters in a clinical trial. Simple blinding means the patient isn't aware if they are taking the drug/therapy or a placebo. In double blinding, the researcher/investigator also won't know which group the patient is in.

Cardinal values

Cardinal refers to a basic or primary value. Examples of cardinal numbers are 1, 2, 3 and 4.

Case-control studies

A study that compares two groups of people: those with the disease or condition under study (cases) and a very similar group of people who do not have the disease or condition (controls). Researchers study the medical and lifestyle histories of the people in each group to learn what factors may be associated with the disease or condition. For example, one group may have been exposed to a particular substance that the other was not.

Clinical effectiveness

The application of interventions which have been shown to be efficacious to appropriate patients in a timely fashion to improve patients' outcomes and value for the use of resources. (Batstone, G. & Edwards, M. (1996) Achieving clinical effectiveness: just another initiative or a real change in working practice? *British Journal of Clinical Governance*, **1(1)**: 19–21.)

Cohort studies

A study in which a particular outcome is monitored over time. An example could be death from a heart attack, when compared to groups of people who are alike in most ways but differ by a certain specific characteristic, for example, smoking.

Cost and Opportunity cost

The economic definition of cost (also known as opportunity cost) is the value of the opportunity forgone (strictly the *best* opportunity forgone), as a result of engaging resources in an activity. Note that there can be a cost without the exchange of money. Also the economists' notion of cost extends beyond the cost falling on the health service alone. For example, it includes costs falling on other services and on patients themselves.

Costs may be considered as follows:

- **Average costs** – the total costs divided by the total number of units.

- **Fixed costs** – those costs which, within a short time span, do not vary with the quantity of production; e.g. heating and lighting.
- **Incremental costs** – the extra costs associated with an expansion in activity of a given service.
- **Marginal cost** – the cost of producing one extra unit.
- **Total costs** – all costs incurred in the production of a set quantity of service.
- **Variable costs** – those costs which vary with the level of production and are proportional to quantities produced.

When considering health economics as well, costs may be differentiated as follows:

- **Avoided costs** – costs caused by a health problem or illness which are avoided by a health care intervention.
- **Direct costs** – those costs borne by the healthcare system, community and patients' families in addressing the illness.
- **Indirect costs** – mainly productivity losses to society caused by the health problem or disease.

Cost benefit analysis

An economic evaluation in which all costs and consequences of a programme are expressed in the same units, usually money. Cost benefit analysis is not commonly used in health economics.

Cost-effectiveness analysis

An economic evaluation in which the costs and consequences of alternative interventions are expressed as cost per unit of health outcome. Cost-effectiveness analysis is often used to determine technical efficiency; i.e., comparison of costs and consequences of competing interventions for a given patient group within a given budget.

Cost-effectiveness plane

A graphical representation of the concept of incremental cost-effectiveness.

Cost minimization analysis

An economic evaluation in which the consequences associated with the competing interventions are the same and in which only the inputs (that is, the costs) are taken into consideration. The aim is to decide the least costly way of achieving the same outcome. (Donaldson, C., Currie, G. & Mitton, C. (2002) Cost effectiveness analysis in health care: contraindications. *British Medical Journal*, **325**: 891.)

Cost utility analysis

A form of economic study design in which interventions which produce different consequences, in terms of both quantity and quality of life, are expressed as '**utilities**'. The best-known utility measure is the 'quality-adjusted life year' or **QALY**. In this case, competing interventions are compared in terms of cost per utility (cost per QALY). *See also* **Quality-adjusted life year**.

Discounting

A technique which allows the calculation of present values of inputs and benefits which accrue in the future. Discounting is based on a time preference which assumes that individuals prefer to forgo a part of the benefits if they accrue them now, rather than fully in the uncertain future. By the same reasoning, individuals prefer to delay costs rather than incur them in the present. The strength of this preference is expressed by the discount rate which is inserted in economic evaluations.

Disease-specific

Attributes which are associated with a specific disease (e.g. breathlessness for asthma), but not only associated with that disease. A disease-specific questionnaire for asthma wouldn't ask questions on cognitive function, for example.

Effectiveness

The contribution which a treatment makes to individuals' utility or welfare, normally (but not necessarily solely) through better health.

Efficiency

Making the best use of available resources; i.e. getting good value for resources. *See also* **Allocative efficiency** and **Technical efficiency**.

EQ-5D or 'Euroqol 5 dimensions'

EQ-5D is a short, 5 question instrument designed specifically for use as a measure of health outcome. The EQ-5D is applicable to a wide range of health conditions and treatments, and provides a simple descriptive profile of health outcomes and a single index value for health status.

Evidence-based medicine

The conscientious, explicit and judicious use of the current best evidence from clinical care research in making decisions about the care of individual patients.

Generic utility instruments

A questionnaire which can generate utilities for any given health state or condition.

Health economics

The study of how scarce resources are allocated among alternative uses for the care of sickness and the promotion, maintenance and improvement of health, including the study of how healthcare and health-related services, their costs and benefits, and health itself are distributed among individuals and groups in society. World Bank (2001) Health Systems Development: Health Economics [online] (http://go.worldbank.org/RQU0H5VGJ0)

(Health) outcome

In health economics, the term 'outcome' or 'health outcome' is used to describe the result of a health care intervention.

Health technology assessment

Evaluation of biomedical technology in relation to cost, efficacy, utilization, etc., and its future impact on social, ethical, and legal systems.

Hierarchy of evidence

A mechanism for determining which study designs have the most power to predict cause and effect. The highest level of evidence is systematic reviews of RCTs, and the lowest level of evidence is expert opinion and consensus statements.

Incremental cost-effectiveness ratio

The ratio of the difference in the cost of two treatments or alternatives divided by the difference in outcome of the two treatments.

Intention to treat (ITT) analysis

Making use of all the data collected from a randomized controlled trial so that all the patients randomized are accounted for in the final results. Many randomized trials report results as being based on 'intention to treat' even though some patients are not included in the final analysis. This, strictly speaking, would not be an ITT analysis.

Marginal analysis

The evaluation of the change in costs and benefits produced by a change in production or consumption of one unit. It examines the effect of small changes in the existing pattern of health care expenditure in a given setting.

Marginal benefit

The value of benefit derived when output is increased by one unit.

Marginal cost – *see* Cost

Meta-analysis

A statistical technique for combining the findings of two or more clinical trials. It is used most frequently to assess the effectiveness of health care interventions.

Opportunity cost

The notion of cost used in economics. *See also* **Cost**

Published clinical literature

Where the results from clinical trials are made available to the public.

Quality-adjusted life year (QALY)

(1) Units of measure of utility which combine life years gained as a result of health interventions/health care programmes with a judgement about the quality of these life years.

(2) A common measure of health improvement used in cost utility analysis, it measures life expectancy adjusted for quality of life. World Bank (2001) Health Systems Development: Health Economics [online] (http://go.worldbank.org/RQU0H5VGJ0)

Quality of life and Health-related QoL (HRQoL)

The term 'quality of life' is used to evaluate the general wellbeing of individuals and societies.

HRQoL – the impact an illness has on quality of life, including the individual's perception of his or her illness.

Ratings scales

A type of measuring instrument in which responses are rated on a continuum or in an ordered set of categories, with numerical values assigned to each point or category.

Scarcity

A situation in which the needs and wants of an individual or group of individuals exceed the resources available to satisfy them.

Sensitivity analysis

A technique which repeats the comparison between inputs and consequences, varying the assumptions underlying the estimates. In so doing, sensitivity analysis tests the robustness of the conclusions by varying the items around which there is uncertainty.

Short form 36 (SF-36)

The SF-36 is a multi-purpose, short form health survey with only 36 questions. It yields an 8-scale profile of functional health and wellbeing scores as well as psychometrically-based physical and mental health summary measures and a preference-based health utility index. (www.SF-36.org)

Societal perspective

The perspective of society as a whole. Health economic analyses typically take a societal perspective to include all benefits of a programme regardless of who receives them, and all costs regardless of who pays them.

Standard gamble

A technique of generating patient preferences based on decision theory of choices under conditions of uncertainty.

Systematic review

A review in which evidence from scientific studies has been identified, appraised and synthesized in a methodical way according to predetermined criteria.

Technical efficiency

Assesses whether a given output can still be achieved by using less of one input while holding all other inputs constant. *See also* **Cost-effectiveness analysis**.

Threshold incremental cost-effectiveness ratio (ICER)

The ICER at which the decision-making body (Government, hospital) has chosen to be a cost-effective use of resources. Any ICER below this threshold is accepted; any above this, rejected.

Time trade-off

A technique of generating patient preferences by offering a hypothetical decision between choosing shorter survival but at a better health state or a longer survival but at their current (inferior) health state.

Utility and Health utility

Utility is a measure of the preference for, or desirability of, a specific level of health status or specific health outcome. Used by economists to signify the satisfaction accruing to a person from the consumption of a good or service. This concept is applied in healthcare to mean the individual's valuation of their state of wellbeing deriving from the use of healthcare interventions.

Validated

Proven to be effective and reliable at capturing and assessing those variables which the instrument was designed to capture and assess.

Willingness to pay

A technique which aims to assign a value to health benefits by directly eliciting individual preferences from members of the general public. People are asked how much they would be prepared to pay to accrue a benefit or to avoid certain events.

Index

The letter g after a page reference indicates an entry in the Glossary